Mental Wellbeing and
Positive Psychology for
Veterinary Professionals

Mental Wellbeing and Positive Psychology for Veterinary Professionals

A Pre-emptive, Proactive and Solution-based Approach

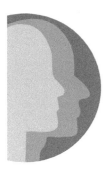

Laura Woodward

WILEY Blackwell

Registered Offices
John Wiley & Sons, Inc., 111 River Street, Hoboken, NJ 07030, USA
John Wiley & Sons Ltd, The Atrium, Southern Gate, Chichester, West Sussex, PO19 8SQ, UK

For details of our global editorial offices, customer services, and more information about Wiley products visit us at www.wiley.com.

Wiley also publishes its books in a variety of electronic formats and by print-on-demand. Some content that appears in standard print versions of this book may not be available in other formats.

Library of Congress Cataloging-in-Publication Data

Names: Woodward, Laura, 1967- author.
Title: Mental wellbeing and positive psychology for veterinary
    professionals : a pre-emptive, proactive and solution-based approach /
    Laura Woodward.
Description: Hoboken, NJ : Wiley-Blackwell, 2024. | Includes index.
Identifiers: LCCN 2023016988 (print) | LCCN 2023016989 (ebook) | ISBN
    9781394200627 (cloth) | ISBN 9781394200634 (adobe pdf) | ISBN
    9781394200641 (epub)
Subjects: MESH: Veterinarians–psychology | Animal Technicians–psychology
    | Mental Health | Psychological Well-Being–psychology | Burnout,
    Professional–prevention & control | Psychology, Positive–methods
Classification: LCC SF745 (print) | LCC SF745 (ebook) | NLM SF 745 | DDC
    636.089092–dc23/eng/20230724
LC record available at https://lccn.loc.gov/2023016988
LC ebook record available at https://lccn.loc.gov/2023016989

Cover Design: Wiley
Cover Images (front and back): Courtesy of Zoe Barr

Set in 9.5/12.5pt STIXTwoText by Straive, Pondicherry, India
Printed and bound by CPI Group (UK) Ltd, Croydon, CR0 4YY

C9781394200627_271123

To my Dad, who loved and believed in me through thick and thin, who proof-read my articles for years, and who laughed with me until the day he died.

To my children Theo and Zoe. Thank you for your encouragement and enthusiasm for this book, your insights and the numerous cups of tea you made for me while I wrote it.

And to Bhante Samitha, who introduced me to mindfulness and meditation, who taught me with compassion and wisdom, and who shares laughter and joy with me at every available opportunity.

Contents

Foreword

Psychological happiness is the ability to maintain a state of peace and contentment whatever life throws at us. It gives us an anchor and a moral compass.

This is not another self-help book for when you are in crisis. This is not something to hand out to your staff like a Band-Aid when they have difficulties. It's designed to be a book for the individual, not a book to be lost amongst the other books on the dusty, groaning practice library shelf.

This is a book designed to help the veterinary workforce to enjoy life with all its twists and turns, using evidence-based methods. This is a pre-emptive and proactive book for when one is happy and wants to help others to thrive. It is for those amongst us who are in difficulty. It is for students prior to qualification, mental health first aiders, for line managers who want to lead with emotional intelligence in a productive way, as well as for those who want to learn about self-care in a career which will definitely challenge them.

This is for people who are happy and want some tools to help others, for people who want to lead from within the team and for those who are contemplating leaving the professions.

Why Are We Here?

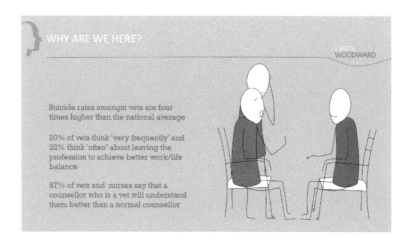

WHY ARE WE HERE?

Laura
WOODWARD

Suicide rates amongst vets are four
times higher than the national average

20% of vets think 'very frequently' and
22% think 'often' about leaving the
profession to achieve better work/life
balance

87% of vets and nurses say that a
counsellor who is a vet will understand
them better than a normal counsellor

Seventy-five percent of vet students wouldn't want anyone to know if they were suffering from a mental health problem, compared to 41% of the general population.
Nearly 39% of vet students have experienced suicidal thoughts.

(above figures from Vet Futures BVA)

Forty-two percent of vets and veterinary nurses have considered leaving the professions.

Vets have four times the national rate of suicide. The suicide rate of veterinary nurses has not been widely reported (the figures shocking in their absence).

There's a pattern here from student to experienced professional.

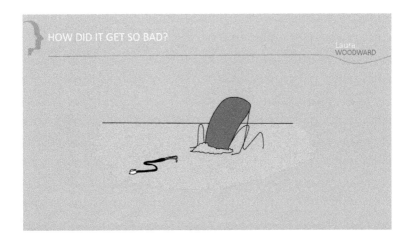

HOW DID IT GET SO BAD?

Laura WOODWARD

Until recently, mental health concerns were taboo in the veterinary world. We have such a 'can do' attitude which we're proud of. It's fantastic that we are physically resilient. We don't take a day off because of a cold, a broken leg or even when we go into labour early.

But is that taking it a bit too far?

'Powering on through' is the way I have worked for decades. If we continue this way, how on earth can our colleagues be open about having depression, anxiety or compassion fatigue?

It is nearly impossible to imagine what depression feels like unless you have suffered from it. Now, as a therapist, I am only just about able to comprehend how debilitating depression and anxiety are. It is harder to get out of bed and go to work when you are depressed than it is to go to work with a broken leg or when in early labour.

If you have never been depressed, you are lucky. Lucky enough to have the strength of mind to realise that you just don't understand how hard it is for some of your close colleagues.

It's okay to not be able to understand. The important thing is to accept that you can't imagine how hard it is.

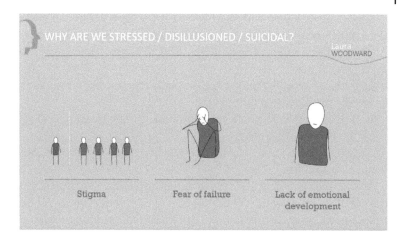

WHY ARE WE STRESSED / DISILLUSIONED / SUICIDAL?

Laura
WOODWARD

Stigma   Fear of failure   Lack of emotional
                                        development

Doing a literature search for hypotheses as to why our professions are in such a state proved fruitless. The reasons will be multifactorial and there will be many differing opinions. My hypothesis is born out of what I have experienced through counselling scores of vets and vet nurses.

Many people in our professions grow up in families that place a big emphasis on achievement, in particular with parents who send mixed messages, alternating between overpraise and criticism. This can increase the risk of fraudulent feelings when we become adults. There can be a lot of confusion between approval and love and worthiness. Self-worth becomes contingent on achieving in these families.

So, as parents, it is our duty to attach our children's self-worth to more than just good grades or medals at football. Kindness is an achievement in kids too. So are empathy, self-regulation, resilience and the ability to be self-aware of our strengths and weaknesses.

Such 'soft skills' fly in the face of 'powering on through'.

But until we realise that true happiness is not solely reliant on social and professional status, we are doing ourselves and our young people a disservice.

I hear similar stories time and time again. Small person is praised for being clever because they can add up two dice in a board game or because they can count to a hundred. They are applauded for being clever, their parents are proud, their grandparents are proud. They get good grades throughout school and their teachers praise them for working so hard.

Achievements follow with maybe a few grade 8s in piano and violin along with grade 9s at GCSEs and A*s at A-level.

They get into vet school or medicine, dentistry or vet nursing and the applause continues.

They are seen as a whole and complete person because of their achievements and they believe it themselves.

But at no stage has anyone stopped to ask if they have good social skills? Do they have empathy?

Do they know how to fail? Or how to fail without falling apart? Do they even know what it feels like?

How are their coping skills for when things go wrong? Have they learnt resilience?

Then comes the workplace. Every day we will all fail to some degree. Usually it's tiny and not to the detriment of our patients. We aim to get it perfect, but we don't always achieve perfection. We have to cope with inexperience and the prospect of getting it wrong and failing. That prospect is paralysing to some new grads.

We need the best social skills of pretty much any profession I know. Loving animals isn't enough. If we don't love people, we'll get stuck because nearly every patient comes with at least one person attached.

We have to have the empathy and social skills to work with these owners, our receptionists, our vets, our nurses, our PCAs, vet students, work experience kids.

New graduate nurses and vets tell me about crippling fear of failure and insomnia. Then they get some more experience and suffer from imposter syndrome: a lonely place to be.

It's exhausting learning social skills and empathy on the job and they suffer from depersonalisation and compassion fatigue. If only they had been taught these soft skills as a child or as a student.

To the leaders and managers, you weren't there when your employees were growing up. But you *are* there now when the new grad turns up or when your student nurses start. Open pre-emptive discussions about mental health, difficulties which will arise, positive psychology, coping tools and tools for joy will be the best welcome gift you can give these employees to help them form cohesive teams and take our professions forward with a determination to be happier and change our god-awful statistics.

> If we were doing enough, doing the right things or doing enough of the right things, our suicide rate would be going down.

What are the major stressors at work?

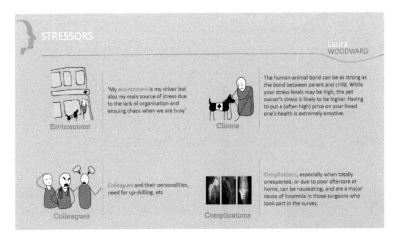

Survey of 40 members of BVOA (British Veterinary Orthopaedic Assoc.) Survey Monkey 2016.

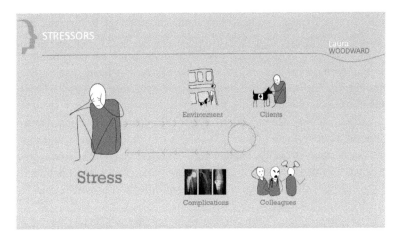

This is a typical day at work for many of us; it's busy or chaotic, our pet owners are understandably stressed or sad and they may pass that onto us, not everything will proceed without complication, there may be people you have to work with who you don't like.

However, it is possible to have the crazy busy day, the difficult clients, the surgical revision and the grumpy colleague and still be happy and joyful. It takes effort and the knowledge of where to place that effort.

How the Book and Ideas Were Developed

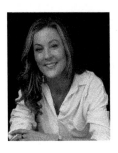 This book has been developed over about six years. For my entire career, I have spent most of my time at work ensconced in the operating theatre with one other person for hours at a time. This 'other person' changes all the time.

As most vets and vet nurses know, there's something about theatre that brings out the deepest of conversations. Maybe it's because the surgeon and the anaesthetist are both masked up and focused on their different tasks rather than facing each other straight on, and we are therefore a bit oblivious to each other's facial reactions to us.

As therapists, we are trained to not face the client directly but rather to sit at an angle to them. It's easier to speak truthfully to someone if you can comfortably avoid eye contact and if you feel you aren't being interrogated. It's the opposite of the interrogation room in any TV cop drama.

Or maybe it's because there's an unwritten rule that what's said in theatre stays in theatre.

I became fascinated with human thoughts and behaviours out of a genuine interest in my colleagues' differing stories.

Then I had children. Their developing minds blew *my* mind, and their learnt and innate behaviours mesmerised me.

I also had adults in my life with difficulties, personality disorders and misbehaviours, as well as other adults who were resilient, compassionate and fun.

This gave me a passion for psychology and I studied to become a counsellor over several years while working.

Because of my children, I specialised in child and adolescent therapy. I then went on to study Buddhist psychotherapy because of the way it looks at our cognitive, energetic and physical being. I love its holistic approach. I also qualified as a mindfulness practitioner and a positive psychologist.

I have been writing for *Veterinary Practice* magazine for over six years and I am very grateful to them for allowing me to use some of the materials I wrote for them in this book.

I still wanted to do more to help to change the mindset of our professions. We are not doing the right things, or enough of the right things, to improve our horrific statistics of mental health crises, burnout and suicide. If we were, the statistics would be improving.

It was after the publication of an article I wrote in Vet Times in 2022 on the neuroscience of suicide that Wiley contacted me to ask me to write this book, and for this I'm also indebted. I have tried to collate all the knowledge I have gleaned from my many mentors, lecturers, leaders and counselling patients over the last decade and place it here in your hands.

I have designed the book to be portable enough to carry around with you, comfortable enough to read in bed, and concise enough that you don't have to go trawling through the internet for some help specific to our professions.

I hope that you will dip in and out of it many times, each time finding something new which applies to you or which you can use to help someone else.

Happiness is not something ready made. It comes from your own actions.

Dalai Lama

How to Use This Book

This edition is designed to be carried around with you, read first thing in the morning and at night-time, dipped into on the bus or train and while at work.

An essential part of any mental health first aider's reading, this book tackles multiple difficulties specific to our veterinary world, and also many others which are part of our often tumultuous life outside work.

Nothing is taboo in this easy-to-follow, gentle but firmly proactive guide to investigating your own emotions and learning to deal with them in a way that works for you.

> *In between a stimulus and our reaction there is a space. In that space lies our freedom to choose our response. Therein lies our freedom.*
> Viktor Frankl

This book will teach you how to recognise the stimulus and how to pause to make the space large enough to choose your own reactions, both internal and external, in order that you'll be happy with your choices. Instead of continuing on autopilot, reacting reflexively and regretting your actions, you will learn to react reflectively in a way which will ultimately make life more enjoyable for you and for those around you.

Part One: Strategies explains effective strategies for dealing with frequent and not so frequent difficulties in our lives, with our multiple roles being taken into consideration and being a reality.

It covers the basics of Mindfulness, Emotional Intelligence, Empathy and so much more, but explained so that we can understand them in a logical fashion and actually apply them in real life today.

This area provides many tools which we will refer to throughout the book. You can skim over it or study it in depth or both. In any case, I hope that you will flip back to it frequently. Some strategies will ring true with some people, and other strategies with other people. You may use one strategy one day and a different strategy with the same situation another time. You are in control of this.

Part Two: How to Meditate: I wrote this in order to demystify the whole process of meditation. Meditation is, of course, another strategy but deserves a whole section to itself.

Meditation can be done at any time, for any length of time, in any place in any clothes. I explain in sensible, effective ways how to incorporate meditation into any hectic life. I understand the many hats we wear as vets, nurses, managers, counsellors, parents, students and family members. Multitasking is part of life. Meditation can also become part of our lives without being the chore at the bottom of the list, and in this section I show the many varied forms which meditation can take.

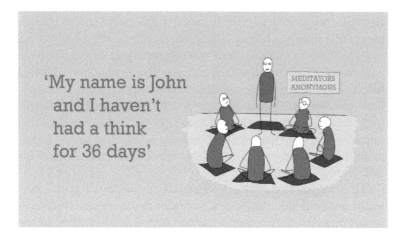

Part Three: Difficulties and Applying Strategies: this is the section to dip in and out of.

Numerous difficulties are discussed here such as anxiety, fear of failure, imposter syndrome, compassion fatigue, grief, burnout and suicide. No one strategy applies to all and so I have suggested tools for you to use in whatever way they work for you here with each difficult topic.

One day, one strategy may help you. Another time, you might want to try a different tool or both. This part *is* self-help. This often makes it more valid for you, and therefore more effective than if you were just doing as instructed.

> The greatest weapon we have against stress is our ability to choose one thought over another.

Part Four: Therapy: Mindfulness is not a panacea and neither are the other strategies. Many of us will benefit from therapy beyond the scope of this book. Part Four explains some of the many therapies available to us and what they entail. It's a minefield until explained. There are differences between CBT, MBSR, ACT, psychotherapeutic counselling, animal-assisted therapy, etc. Here, we simplify and demystify again. Nobody, especially somebody who is overwhelmed and in crisis, should have to blindly figure out the best type of therapy for them.

Part Five: Case Studies: sometimes it's helpful, and also fascinating, to see how others react and behave in different situations with which we are familiar. Part Five uses cases from real counselling sessions (anonymous and altered to protect identities) and sees how they applied different tools to help them navigate the difficulties they brought to the counselling room. We are complex creatures and these cases are brought to life by demonstrating that any crisis is multifactorial. I've never met a client in counselling who had only one problem or only one cause of their problems. These case studies are from vets and vet nurses examining their journeys and the various life-hurdles they met along their paths.

This section can help students, new graduates and recent graduates to see what may lie ahead of them, as I often see these patterns recurring. If we are prewarned of common difficulties, we are less likely to feel shocked and alone when they happen to us. If we are prearmed with a selection of tools to deal with life's difficulties, we won't burn out, leave the profession or take our own lives.

Part Six: Positive Psychology: 'Life is for living' may sound like a meme, but it makes so much sense. Positive psychology is all around us. We no longer buy alarm clocks, we have gentle lights which gradually awake us and then a burst of birdsong greets us to start the day. It's the experience we want, not just the functionality.

My friend's new car greets her when she hops in with a customised seat position and preheated steering wheel. This is the fun world of product design, realising that we want to have pleasant experiences, not to just 'get through it'.

Mental wellbeing can learn from this, and this last part of the book suggests ways for us to promote our experience from okay to good, from good to great or from great to fantastic. This is not beyond our reach, nor is it selfish. If we achieve a level of bonhomie which we can spread around us, and create an aura of calm and wellbeing even for just a few minutes of each day, we make the world a better place.

> Just one breath, taken mindfully, can change the course of our day. A few days like that and we can change the course of our life, if we choose.

Part 1

Strategies

Mindfulness

- What does 'mindfulness' mean?
- Mindful living
- Mindfulness: how to do it
- An introduction to mindful meditation
- The case for mindfulness versus I'm already too busy
- Mindfulness in the veterinary practice
- Mindfulness and management

What Does 'Mindfulness' Mean?

Jon Kabat Zinn, a very well-known mindfulness teacher and advocate, defines mindfulness as 'paying attention to the present moment on purpose, non-judgementally'.

Paying Attention to the Present Moment

It's so hard to make ourselves aware of 'just now' for an extended period of time. Our minds naturally wander to tasks that need to be done, things we need to sort out, what happened last night, what may happen next weekend, who just walked in, the cat needs feeding, my phone's beeping, etc.

Non-judgement

Begins with awareness of your own thoughts and stopping yourself from labelling any of them as good or bad. But how can we do this?

> *Everything can be taken from a man but one thing: the last of the human freedoms – to choose one's attitude in any given set of circumstances.*
>
> Viktor E. Frankl

Take a moment to examine whether you are the type of person to see an event and then reflexively judge it as 'right' or 'wrong'? Or do you hear about someone, see their Facebook post and jump to a 'good' or 'bad' conclusion? It's okay if you do. Most of us do just that.

Mental Wellbeing and Positive Psychology for Veterinary Professionals: A Pre-emptive, Proactive and Solution-based Approach, First Edition. Laura Woodward.
© 2024 John Wiley & Sons Ltd. Published 2024 by John Wiley & Sons Ltd.

People bitching about other people is designed to sway our judgements of the person being talked about. Do you side with the slanderer? Are you easily swayed? Do you feel obliged to pass judgement even if you don't act upon it? It's human nature.

Politicians try to sway us into judgement as their full-time job. Celebrities, news channels, Instagram all ask us to judge. And we do. Now imagine what it would be like if you consciously chose not to judge any more. What a weight is lifted off your shoulders if you decide you don't have to take sides, pass judgement, make decisions about who's right and who's wrong.

It starts off as a conscious decision. With a little time, it becomes part of you. It is the most liberating feeling of relief when you make a conscious decision to not get involved in all the judging of others. I advise you to try it for one day or even one hour and then spend some time contemplating how it feels for you.

Mindful Living

This can be done literally anywhere, at any time, for a few seconds, for a whole day, or as a permanent thing. It still involves focusing on the present moment on purpose non-judgmentally, with curiosity and awe as if we had never noticed it before. It can also include time sitting on the cushion. The point is that it really is attainable for anyone. With practice, it rapidly becomes your personal way of being.

And all of this can be incorporated into your hectic daily schedule without losing any of your time.

In the book *Skills Training Manual for Treating Borderline Personality Disorder*, Marsha Linehan describes one such way of bringing yourself to the present moment by using the mindfulness skill called 'observe'. Observe is about merely noticing what is happening right now. It is just noticing – nothing more. Often it can be more powerful to just notice the present rather than think about the present. Seeing with fresh eyes in a non-judgemental way like a child can be liberating and a breath of fresh air for your frazzled mind. You can try that right now. It really is just a snapshot commentary of 'now' to bring you into the present moment. For example "I'm sitting on the bed reading a book on mental wellbeing". What's the point of this? Probably the easiest way to answer that is to recommend you try it a few times today and see what it feels like for you.

George de Mestral was a Swiss engineer in the 1940s. He was known to be a bit of a genius. What is less known about him is that he kept his mind sharp by taking regular breaks in nature, walking mindfully. So, while many of us might walk the dog while catching up on Facebook, or go for a run to clear our heads, get some steps in and get fitter, only to be disappointed that our minds are still cluttered at the end, George would walk painstakingly slowly, noticing all the different shades of green (42 apparently), the shape of the trees, the shape of the leaves on the trees, the shape of the veins on the leaves on the trees, and so on.

Well, George noticed the hooks on the seeds of the trees so closely, with awe and wonder, that he invented Velcro and never had to work again.

Jon Kabat Zinn asks in a famous interview with Oprah, 'When you're in the shower, are you actually *in the shower*?' It's a poignant question. I shamefully put my hand up and say that I'm usually not in the shower when I'm 'in the shower'. I'm triaging the day's tasks, I'm planning my surgical list, I'm thinking about what the kids need for school and what I'm going to make for dinner.

But I know for sure that if I left this plethora of thoughts outside the shower, it would be so good for me. If I, or you, spent 10 minutes getting up earlier and doing our triage list, then hopped into the shower and focused on the present moment, the temperature, the sound and feel of the water, the scent of the shower gel and the gratitude we feel for having all these luxuries, we would benefit enormously from it.

And we wouldn't even have started meditation yet. Try it once. It will be difficult. Don't judge yourself if your mind strays. Then try it again.

Habituation

Our brains are designed to stop us paying too much attention. This is well demonstrated by the optical illusion called Troxler fading (named after the nineteenth-century Swiss physician who discovered the effect). If presented with a steady image in the area of our peripheral vision, we actually stop seeing it after a while. This phenomenon – the general neuroscientific term is **habituation** – probably points to an efficient way in which the brain operates. Neurons stop firing once they have sufficient information about an unchanging stimulus. But this does not mean that habituation is always our friend.

We can consider the effort not just to think differently but also to see differently as a way of countering our built-in tendency to habituate – to sink into the familiar way of seeing and experiencing. By running on autopilot, we are in danger of missing out on the sheer, unadulterated pleasure we can get from the fact that a seemingly mundane, boring thing is actually running to plan. It may be an unchanging stimulus and yet be a potential source of joy for us if we allow it to be noticed.

It's all too easy to divert our attention to problems or malfunctions and miss out on the times when everything is actually and beautifully okay.

The great French mathematician Blaise Pascal said: 'Small minds are concerned with the extraordinary, great minds with the ordinary'.

Mindfulness: How to Do It

Mindfulness can be anything from taking a moment to appreciate a beautiful view, to taking a few deep breaths, to mini-meditations, to full meditation in cross-legged posture for an hour or more every day.

> No act is better or worse than the others. What matters is that you choose what works for you.

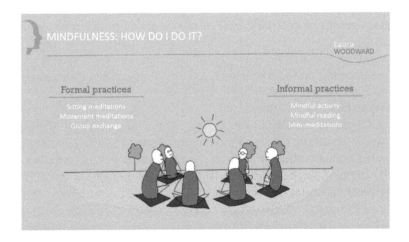

Incorporating mindfulness into your life can be done in any way you choose.

Formal Mindfulness Practices

Formal practices might be an easy way to start if you want guidance at the beginning. When I go to the gym, I love classes where the teacher does all the motivation and I just have to do what I'm told as energetically as I can. Similarly, guided meditation or other guided practices teach and motivate us.

Unguided meditation and other practices often have a more powerful effect and you can tailor them to your own needs. So while mindfulness apps and YouTube meditations are a fantastic place to start, I urge you to move on to unguided as your norm or as an adjunct to your practice as soon as you feel you can.

Sitting meditations can be for three minutes or three hours and anything in between. Sitting upright is important; this is not about being in a daze, it's about being more acutely alert and awake than ever before.

Movement meditation is a very serene mindfulness practice. Mindful walking involves walking so slowly that you notice every part of your foot as it gradually takes one step and then every part of the other foot as it gradually moves through its step, all the while feeling gratitude for the solid ground, our ability to move and having the time to appreciate what we normally take for granted through habituation.

Group exchange in Buddhism is called *Sangha*, where a community of friends gather together to practise the dharma (the teachings of the Buddha) together, to bring about and maintain awareness. Being in a group talking about mindfulness, or the dharma, or in Alcoholics Anonymous, gives people strength and encouragement to persevere towards their common goals. Knowing that you are amongst like-minded people, even if there is only one thing you all have in common, is comforting and opens us up to new ways of thinking.

Informal Mindfulness Practices

Informal mindfulness practices may include a mindful activity. There is a bottomless list of opportunities to do this every day. Mindful cooking involves taking more time than I want to make a meal. I'm usually aiming for the best meal in the shortest time possible. However, on the days where I decide to do this task slowly and mindfully, it's a pleasure. Lots of people glean enormous amounts of pleasure from cooking. Others adore cooking programmes and there is a plethora of cooking and baking programmes to watch on TV. So there has to be something in this mindful cooking lark.

Taking the ingredients and noticing things about them which we haven't taken the time to notice before is a good place to start. Feeling the ingredients, smelling them, listening to the sound of them being cut might sound comical and we can have so much fun with this. It *is* comical and therein lies the humour because mindfulness isn't about being straight-faced and strait-laced sitting cross-legged on a painful cushion.

Noticing aromas, textures and flavours, feeling grateful that we have a fridge, home delivery and the cash to enjoy both is a simple gratitude practice we can use while cooking.

Mowing the lawn is one of my favourites. The smell of freshly cut grass means that spring or summer is here. I love growing a lawn. I'm grateful to not have hay fever. I can take this hour out of my weekend to make geometrical parallel stripes on my lawn with a roller. I can look out of my window and admire those stripes several times a day afterwards in all types of changing daylight.

Mindful activity is about being present in the moment and noticing in a child-like wondorous way using all of our senses. It is the opposite of mindless activity and distraction techniques.

Mindful reading usually involves a carefully chosen text which is designed to provoke thought. For example, it may be a text which we can dip in and out of, read a short passage and then sit in quiet contemplation about that passage and what it means to us personally. It could be this book or another book with many small thought-provoking passages, etc.

Mindful reading might be reading poetry slowly and noticing how we see different things each time we read it, looking at photo books or books about paintings.

I have a book by my bed with 365 different mindful practices, one for each day of the year. When I am having trouble focusing during meditation, one passage from this book rescues me and gives something to contemplate.

An Introduction to Mindful Meditation

This will be a recurring theme in this book and I've dedicated a whole section to how to meditate (see Part Two).

Mindfulness and meditation are inextricably linked so it's worth demystifying meditation briefly at this point, especially as we'll be dipping in and out of the book in random fashion as you please.

Mini-meditations are what we're doing often without realising. Mini means as small as you want. If you take three deep breaths while waiting for an elevator to arrive, that is a mini-meditation. So you're probably doing this already in some shape or form. It isn't hard and it doesn't take up any valuable time in our hectic veterinary roles.

> Only you can meditate for you.

Mindful meditation is only one part of living mindfully. Meditation can have profound effects on those who subscribe to doing it habitually. If we can make it part of our daily routine, the results can be life changing.

I was sceptical too. And yet almost as soon as I discovered how powerful mindful meditation is (and it works immediately), I was sold.

Although mindfulness as a concept has been around for thousands of years, its application in Western psychology is relatively recent.

Meditation will help you discover an understanding of how thoughts and feelings influence your behaviour.

A word of caution from personal experience: although the beneficial effects are immediate, which is very rewarding and incentivising, if you skip a morning or two, there are no residual benefits from the meditation you did last week. It has to become a daily habit to change every day for the better.

And I suppose that is a no-brainer. If we are truly living in the moment, on purpose, then it is fitting that the meditation we do today affects us today.

Also, there is a huge difference between non-guided meditation, which we are aiming for here, and guided meditation which can be done using apps, etc. While any meditation is better than none, the benefits of unguided over guided meditation are enormous. It takes so much more time to achieve the same results with an app than it does if you are your own guide.

Mindful Meditation: Paying Attention, on Purpose

If you've been meditating for some time already, well done. Sometimes it can be useful to bring yourself back to the basics of pinpoint concentration on 'nothingness'. See how long you can manage that for. It takes enormous focus and discipline to be able to maintain this clarity of mind. It is so important to start any meditation session clarifying the mind like this.

For those embarking on meditation for the first time, it may be too difficult to focus on nothing. I advise beginners to focus on 'something' instead. For example, try focusing on your breath and nothing else. It doesn't have to be deep breaths or shallow. It can be any breaths you take. Notice it. See if you can maintain focus on your breathing and on nothing else. If that's not working for you, some people find it useful to count the breaths to maintain focus.

All thoughts that try to enter your mind at this stage, you need to gently push aside. Right here, right now, you are clearing your mind and all thoughts can wait until another time. By 'creating extra time' in your day, you deserve these moments to not be organising/sorting/thinking. If you hadn't set the alarm to meditate, you wouldn't be sorting them out either, you'd be asleep, so they just have to wait until later.

If you do find that your mind has wandered, it isn't failure. Rather, it's useful that you notice it. Each time you gently push those thoughts to the left or to the right, you are getting better at clearing your mind. It takes training to become good at maintaining the focus.

Some people imagine a narrow slit of light in front of them. This light is the clear mind they are aiming for. As each thought enters their mind, they push it to the left or right as if pushing back the shutters to open their mind and make this slit of light wider and wider until it becomes a window of light to focus on.

One practitioner I met started his meditations with reciting the words 'just' at every inhalation and 'now' at each exhalation until he achieved total focus.

Whatever works for you is great.

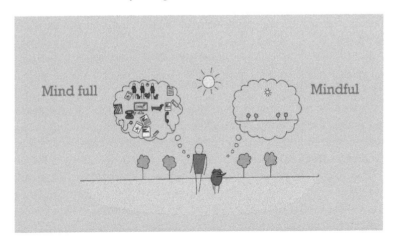

So my mind is clear. Big deal. Now what?

It's hard for me to describe just how much maintaining clarity of mind for extending periods of time can make an average day feel fantastic. Our worries about the future and past can negatively influence our behaviour in the present. Mindfulness potentially counters this process by teaching us to focus on the current moment.

For this month, achieving a clear mind each morning for as long as you possibly can is enough.

Observe if you find it easier as the weeks go by.

Notice if some mornings it's easier than others.

> Instead of waiting endlessly for the perfect time to start a daily mindfulness practice, we could instead just start.

Mindful Meditation: Non-judgement of Emotions

So during your morning meditation session, now that we are *au fait* with achieving clarity of the mind for extended periods of time, it's a perfect time to allow our emotions to envelop us. It takes discipline and inner strength to allow the emotions which have previously been overwhelming to come to the forefront of our mind one by one.

Self-awareness means being acutely alert and aware of what we're feeling. This is *not* about burying emotions in a box and ignoring them. It is about being actively aware of these emotions, however distressing or otherwise they may be, and feeling them one by one, so that the full force of the emotion is there. Then, and only then, can we defuse it, if we wish.

Give one emotion a name, look it in the face, allow it to envelop you and accept that you are feeling what you are feeling. The more you accept and embrace that emotion, the more you defuse it and decrease its power over you.

Now the non-judgement. . . Non-judgement begins with awareness of your own thoughts and stopping yourself from labelling any of them as good or bad. They just are. Accept your thoughts and feelings as natural and allow them to come.

Non-reacting is the skill of allowing your thoughts and feelings to be, without resorting to the need to behave reactively in the same way you have reacted before. No one ever healed from a blow to the head by hitting themselves there again.

Pause for a moment to reflect on your inner experience. Don't act hastily and emotionally.

> *Between stimulus and response there is a space. In that space is our power to choose our response. In our response lies our growth and our freedom.*
>
> Viktor E. Frankl

So now, you can make this space as large as you like. And you can literally choose how you want to react to this emotion internally as well as externally. What you choose to do in your morning meditation, you will do subconsciously later in the day.

Let's consider a couple of frequent emotions we can approach in this way with an open mind. We will use anger and anxiety many times in this book.

Anger

For example, if I feel angry, I feel angry. Having the emotion is not good nor bad. It is what it is.

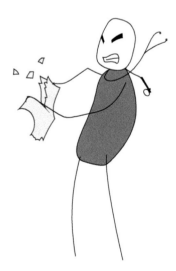

There may be many reasons why I am angry and the causes of how I'm feeling right now are in the past. Maybe the causes will never stop but the way I feel right now is a result of what has happened up to this point, and the past cannot be changed or undone.

Right now, while allowing the anger to envelop me, I have a choice to make. Would I like the internal reaction to be 'to feel less angry'? Is it a sign of weakness that the same things/people which caused the anger will remain the same and I am changing to be less reactive?

Does that mean that I'm allowing them to 'win'? Or, in choosing to suffer less, am I indeed being responsibly selfish enough to be the 'winner'?

That's for you to answer.

> *Pain is inevitable. Suffering is optional.*
>
> Dalai Lama

But if your motivation is to feel less hate, less hypertension and less pain, then maybe you will choose to simply feel less preoccupied and less consumed by the anger when the stimulus occurs next time. It is genuinely a choice.

Or maybe the cause of the anger is gone, in which case it's even easier to simply feel less anger about the past from now on. If that's what you choose.

No matter how justified your anger is, if you choose to let the feelings of rage go, then you may feel *more* empowered and *more* free than the perpetrator if you choose to defuse it.

Once the internal reaction has been chosen, what do I want my external reaction to be? Again that's your choice. Maybe you want to send an eloquent email. Maybe you feel that throwing furniture is appropriate. Maybe you want to try something new if the previous external actions haven't achieved an optimal result. Maybe you want to try (dare I suggest it) showing compassion towards an adversary.

It may be that, once the internal rage has become so weak that it's way down your list of priorities now, your external reaction is naturally one of calmness and physical non-reactivity in the face of what would have previously enraged you.

> Holding onto distressing and painful emotions disempowers you. Letting go of them, if that's what you choose, relieves the stress and burden on you to feel responsible for everything, especially those things that you cannot change.

Anxiety

Anger is just one emotion which can be looked at in this way. Anxiety is a great emotion to work with in a similar step-by-step fashion. Fear, grief and regret may be on your list also. When embracing anxiety and feeling it to its full extent, it can be quite nauseating and stressful. You may find your stomach sinking, your pulse increasing, your breaths becoming gasps. 'Letting go' of anxiety is simply too difficult and impractical for most people due to its biochemical aspects as well as the external causes.

Spending extended periods of time focusing on 'nothingness' can help with anxiety, as can breathing meditations where you focus on your breaths and nothing else for as long as possible (ideally 20 minutes at a time). It's so hard but it's so effective.

However, probably the most powerful tool I have used with my clients, along with the above, is learning to accept that anxiety is not going to go away any time soon. Acceptance of anxiety as a part of your life (if it is), which contrasts so profoundly with trying to make it go away or cure it, can feel like lying down passively and succumbing to the horrors of it all. However, if fighting against anxiety hasn't worked this far, and 'letting go' of anxiety is simply too difficult, maybe allowing it to just be, to play along in the background and be accepted for what it is, will decrease its hold over you.

Hans Selye said: 'It's not stress that kills us. It's our reaction to it'.

The Case for Mindfulness versus I'm Already Too Busy

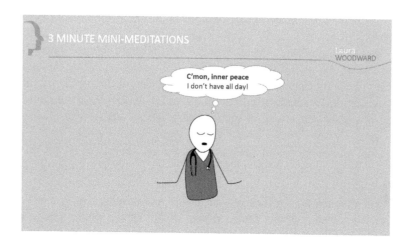

Paying attention to the present moment on purpose, non-judgementally.

It's so hard to make ourselves aware of 'just now' for an extended period of time. Our minds naturally wander to tasks that need to be done, things we need to sort out, what happened last night, what may happen next weekend, etc.

At work, we focus on problem lists, the consults coming in next, the ops list, the bad debts, the complaints not yet dealt with. Rarely do we take the time to focus on the here and now. It's a luxury enjoyed by few. We don't have the time. I never focus on the surgeries that went right. They don't need my energy and attention any more so why should I? The hundreds of happy clients don't take up as much headspace as the one complaint letter or surgical complication.

But mindfulness isn't all about sitting cross-legged on the cushion in a meditative state focusing on the present for an hour. Maybe you're a member of the early morning lot who wake up at 5 a.m. to meditate. Maybe it suits you to be mindful while in a yoga session.

What isn't helpful is for you to berate yourself for not managing to find the time to 'be better' at mindfulness. It's about being non-judgmental, remember?

No Time to Meditate

In its purest and most effective form, deep meditation is often pin-point concentration on nothingness for a period of time to calm the chaotic mind.

You need to literally 'make time' for this. Usually, the best time for meditation is upon waking. How often is frantically scrolling through your phone the first thing you do in the day? On top of this rapid input of information needing to be processed, our minds usually are at their most chaotic and disorganised the moment we wake up. What a stressful way to start our days.

For those embarking on meditation for the first time, it may be too difficult to focus on nothing. I advise beginners to focus on 'something' instead.

For example, try *focusing on your breath* and nothing else. Notice it. See if you can maintain focus on your breathing and nothing else. If that's not working for you, some people find it useful to count the breaths to maintain focus. If it's still too difficult, try putting your hand over your heart and feel your chest rise and fall with the breaths. This is very much in the present moment.

All thoughts which try to enter your mind at this stage, you need to gently push aside. Right here, right now, you are clearing your mind and all thoughts can wait until another time. By creating extra time in your day, you deserve these moments to be spent *not* organising, sorting or thinking. If you hadn't set the alarm to meditate, you wouldn't be sorting them out either – you would be asleep – so they just have to wait until later.

If you do find that your mind has wandered, it isn't failure. Rather, it is useful that you notice it. Remember the non-judgement? Each time you gently push those thoughts to the left or the right, you are getting better at clearing your mind. It takes training to become good at maintaining the focus.

> Even if you do this for only five minutes a day, every day, it will change your life.

Many people need *guided meditation* to give them a commentary or they will be distracted. This is not failure. It's noticing, non-judgementally, their need for what is right for them. YouTube has a massive choice. The

HealthyMinds app has lessons as well as meditations on a range of areas, such as insight and purpose, of whatever length you choose. The lessons are great to listen to on your commute.

Non-judgement

What does that mean? Non-judgement is accepting your experiences, thoughts and feelings instead of judging them to be 'right' or 'wrong', 'justified' or 'bad', etc.

> No one ever healed a blow to the head by hitting themselves there again.

By that, I mean that if you are already feeling what you deem to be a 'wrong' emotion, e.g. anger at someone, you are unlikely to defuse its hold on you by then judging yourself as a bad person for having the feeling and being angry with yourself in addition.

Non-judgement isn't just about judging or not judging ourselves or other people. It's about allowing *emotions* to flow without feeling the obligation to 'fix' them. It's about noticing *experiences*, pleasant and unpleasant, without yearning for things to be different and wishing they hadn't happened.

Once you relieve yourself of the full-time job of placing everything into 'good' or 'bad' categories, it can feel like a huge weight has been lifted off your shoulders.

How to Start (Ironically at the End)

There is no shame in starting mindfulness in a tiny and easy way.

Take one breath in and out, notice you are doing it and finish with the word 'yes' (as in 'yes I did that'). That, done a few times a day, is a worthwhile place to start.

Mindfulness in the Veterinary Practice

How can we work more mindfully in the practice and why should we aim for that?

These are valid questions especially when we are quite reliant on our leaders and managers implementing a new way of working. The old jaded methods are exactly that: old-fashioned.

Everything we do has to be evidence based and that's a great thing. The evidence base for mindfulness is littered throughout this book with references I urge you to explore.

One source of evidence suggesting that the surgical team simply must work mindfully is a book by an American human surgeon, Atul Gwande: *The Checklist*. Atul was already a successful surgeon when the World Health Organization approached him and asked him how surgeons could reduce morbidity and mortality. What a difficult question to answer.

At this time, the volume of surgery was increasing rapidly but the safety of surgery was not. Usually, the normal protocol would be to introduce more training or more technology to improve outcomes, but this had already been done to minimal avail. The US surgeons were already highly trained, yet overall mortality from all surgery in the States was at 1.5% and surgical complications at 11%.

Atul interviewed highly trained individuals from other industries such as pilots and skyscraper engineers and asked them what they had that surgeons didn't? They had the technology and the training but they also had checklists.

Checklists are tools to help make experts better.

We've all seen pilots and co-pilots run through checklists on TV and in real life; engineers have to do the same or the skyscraper will bend.

Atul approached a leading safety engineer at Boeing to ask if they could help him to devise a safety checklist for surgical teams. Designing a checklist to handle complexity is difficult. He came up with a few drafts where the checklist would identify 'pause points', i.e. moments to catch a problem before it becomes a danger.

The end-product was a 19-item, two-minute checklist focusing on key items which can get missed. It included team members introducing themselves by first name and role in order to make the team more cohesive during that procedure and ready to deal with incidents as they arise. This introduction is an ice breaker in a way. It also removes the hierarchical tone which can cause confusion if there is a crisis.

To test this checklist, it was implemented in a large selection of hospitals all over the world. To make the results more valid, hospitals were chosen at random and included those in affluent areas and countries as well as those in third-world countries and areas of poverty.

The results were shocking. Using this checklist resulted in a 35% decrease in surgical complications and a 47% decrease in surgical mortality across the board.

And yet there was resistance to introducing the routine use of checklists in many hospitals. Why? Probably because it's hard to confront what we're not used to. We're used to doing things as we've always done them, and the fear of change brings the fear of decreasing our abilities as surgeons and anaesthetists. It's hard to accept that we are not a faultless system.

When it comes to indications for a particular surgical approach, technique or protocol, often 'surgeon preference' is the indication, i.e. to stay with what we're comfortable with and experienced with. Yet, we also have to keep up with evidence-based studies which might be telling us to change our methods.

It was difficult to encourage surgical teams to embrace different values, e.g. humility, discipline, team work, etc., especially if they had previously been guided by a lead surgeon whose first name was unknown.

However, now surgical checklists are the norm and we rarely question their usage. Two minutes to drastically pre-empt morbidity and mortality cannot be argued with.

At the start, we introduce ourselves (sometimes awkwardly because we've known each other for decades) by our first name and our role in that procedure.

The pause points are before general anaesthesia, before incision and before leaving the OR, and can include:

- the patient's full name correlating with their neck tag
- the procedure being undertaken and which has been authorised by the owner
- the limb/side, etc. of the procedure
- the possible complications envisaged during the procedure
- the availability and sterility of blood, fluids, equipment, etc.
- the anaesthetic and analgesic agents being used
- the swab and sharps counts prior to incision, during the surgery and at closure
- the samples taken and what tests will be conducted on them
- the immediate postoperative plan for the patient.

These checklists can be tailored to our individual clinics

So what does a checklist have to do with mindfulness at work? Well, it is actually a form of mindfulness because it forces us to stop, focus and be completely present. Focusing 100% on our patient and their procedure not only makes good clinical sense, it serves us and our colleagues well in all the ways other forms of mindfulness do. When we are totally engrossed in our task instead of trying to remember to return phone calls, look at CT scans and interpret blood results all at the same time, we can be calmer, less frazzled and achieve a better outcome.

It takes only two minutes a few times a day to achieve all of this.

Mindfulness and Management

See Chapter 24 in Part Three: Mindfulness as an evidence-based tool to prevent stress, burnout and depersonalisation.

The case for mindfulness is so strong that for HR not to promote it as part of the workplace culture is to miss a real opportunity to optimise patient care by promoting clinician self-care.

Emotional Intelligence

- The five competencies of emotional intelligence
- Self-awareness
- Self-regulation
- Motivation
- Empathy
- Social skills

The Five Competencies of Emotional Intelligence

Daniel Goleman is known by some as the father of emotional intelligence but what is it?

> Emotional intelligence is the ability to perceive, control and evaluate emotions in yourself and in others.

What does that look like? There are five competencies of emotional intelligence described by Daniel Goleman.

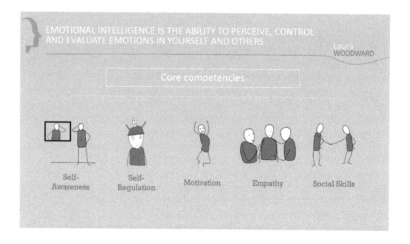

Mental Wellbeing and Positive Psychology for Veterinary Professionals: A Pre-emptive, Proactive and Solution-based Approach, First Edition. Laura Woodward.
© 2024 John Wiley & Sons Ltd. Published 2024 by John Wiley & Sons Ltd.

1) *Self-awareness* is the ability to be introspective to such a degree as to recognise the emotions within us at the present time, emotions from the past and also the emotions we are likely to feel in a given situation in the future. We are aware of our strengths and our limitations. We are also aware of past behaviours which have followed on from certain emotions.

2) *Self-regulation*: when emotions are running high, they certainly cannot be ignored – but they can be carefully managed. This is called self-regulation, and it's the quality of emotional intelligence that liberates us from living like hostages to our impulses.

3) *Motivation*: what do I want out of a given situation and how can I achieve it?
   Being 'responsibly selfish'.

4) *Empathy*: the ability to see things from another's perspective. This is so important, even if you don't agree with the other perspective, that I have dedicated a whole chapter to its various forms (see Chapter 3, Part One).

5) *Social skills*: without good communication skills, the ability to actively listen and make eye contact with each other, to verbalise eloquently and use our body language effectively, we may as well be dogs in the park with only a tail for communication (if we're lucky).

If your emotional abilities aren't in hand, if you don't have self-awareness, if you are not able to manage your distressing emotions, if you can't have empathy and have effective relationships, then no matter how smart you are, you are not going to get very far.

Daniel Goleman

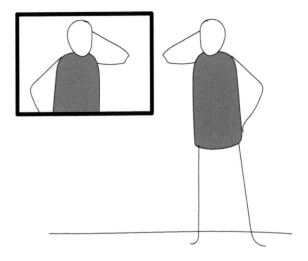

Self-awareness

Described by Daniel Goleman as the foundation of emotional intelligence, self-awareness is the ability to be introspective to such a degree as to recognise the emotions within us at the present time, emotions from the past and also the emotions we are likely to feel in a given situation in the future. We are aware of our strengths and our limitations. We are also aware of past behaviours which have followed on from certain emotions.

Being non-judgemental is an essential but difficult part of self-awareness. If we see certain emotions as 'good' or 'bad', then observing them can become uncomfortable for us.

> To have disturbing emotions is human. To err is also human. However, to err repeatedly in the same way in reaction to these emotions is entirely within our control. This is self-regulation.

If ignored, behaviours and reactions to feelings generally repeat themselves and we can become conditioned to react in a certain way each time we feel a particular emotion.

Spending our lives in denial and in ignorance of our deeper selves will inevitably result in repetition of those behaviours which have led to our distress in the first place. For example, fear of failure may lead to anxiety, anger may lead to shouting and alienation of loved ones or colleagues, grief may lead to depression.

However, we cannot begin to self-regulate if we lack true self-awareness. So, try not to judge yourself for feeling a feeling. There are plenty of people who will do that job for you!

By all means do judge your reactions. Self-regulation is our moral compass and the second competency of emotional intelligence.

How Do I Become More Self-aware?

Daniel Kahneman, who won a Nobel Prize for his contribution to behavioural science, talked about the difference between the experiencing self and the remembering self, and how it can affect our decision making. He explains that how we *feel* about the experience in the moment and how we *remember* the experience can be very different and share only 50% correlation. And this difference can have a significant impact on the story we are telling ourselves, the way we relate to self and others, and the decisions we make, even though we may not notice the difference most of the time.

Being Aware of Present Self

Be mindful. Pay attention to your inner state all day and try to make observing it the new normal for you. We have discussed how to practise mindfulness and being focused on the present in Chapter 1. If done daily, we are observing our thoughts as they happen, rather than trying to remember them days or weeks later.

When Overwhelmed

Take time to look inwards at the gamut of emotions you may be feeling at times when your head is spinning. Write them down one by one. Practise the conveyor belt meditation in Part Two, Chapter 4.

Simply by recognising each emotion, acknowledging it and giving it a name, we can take more charge of our emotions and thus more control of our ensuing reactions. It puts us in charge of our feelings rather than our feelings being our master.

Once you have written the emotions down, arrange them in order of importance. A triage list. Once 'sorted', you may feel less overwhelmed and in a better place to observe whether you have any conditioned behaviours related to these emotions which you would like to change.

Once focused, then we truly have the power to change our reactions to given situations. Simply being aware of our previous conditioned reactions gives us the option to continue with that behaviour or to reject it in favour of a more productive behaviour. It's your choice and entirely under your control.

Self-regulation

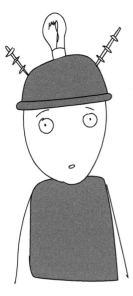

When emotions are running high, they certainly cannot be ignored – but they can be carefully managed. This is called **self-regulation** and it's the quality of emotional intelligence that liberates us from living like hostages to our impulses.

We're now aware of the concept of self-awareness, i.e. being in touch with our emotions and also our conditioned responses to those emotions. By being self-regulatory, we can choose how we want to respond to those emotions and take control of our responses both external and (importantly to our wellbeing) internal.

People who have high levels of emotional intelligence are less likely to respond instantaneously and reactively to a difficult or challenging situation. Allowing your reflexes to determine your actions can often lead to ongoing distressing emotions and a rollercoaster of emotional turmoil.

> *Compassion and tolerance are not signs of weakness, but signs of strength.*
> Dalai Lama

The response of a person with good levels of self-regulation is the response which that person has consciously chosen to have. For example, when that work colleague chooses to rant at me, I can allow the chain of pain, low self-esteem, bad-mouthing and insomnia to take hold once again. Or I can choose to:

- recognise the pain from the insult, non-judgementally, and allow myself to feel it and own it
- place the insult firmly in the past, and
- stop the chain of unhelpful subsequent conditioned responses to it right there.

Every time you do this, it helps to make it the 'new normal' response, and with time, it will become the conditioned response to the inevitable ranting of the emotionally unintelligent colleague.

People with high running emotional intelligence are likely to have:

- an inclination towards *reflection and thoughtfulness*
- *an acceptance of uncertainty* and change
- *integrity* – specifically the ability to say 'no' to impulsive urges.

Reflection and Thoughtfulness

This is our mindfulness practice in the chapters on how to meditate. If we spend only 10 minutes mindfully meditating every day, self-awareness and self-regulation become easier. If you spend an hour a day, they become an integral part of you.

Acceptance of Uncertainty and Change

The world is ever-changing. Our lives are ever-changing. What we think of as a 'given' in our lives can be snatched from us suddenly with devastating effects if we are not open to change. We desperately cling onto our status quo and yet our parents die and our partners cheat. No two days are the same.

Change can be unsettling, big changes can be distressing and bereavement can lead to relentless grief. We have to work at accepting it. The emotionally intelligent person finds self-regulation easier because they embrace the unexpected no matter how good or bad it is.

Integrity and the ability to say 'no' to impulsive urges are important. If we are truly compassionate, if we are self-aware and if we have good morals, then we are less likely to give in to impulsive urges such as the urgent need to blame someone or something for every unpleasant event in our lives. Narcissistic people often justify blaming others for their own unhappiness in a very convincing way, usually easily convincing themselves at the same time.

The emotionally intelligent, self-regulating person doesn't need to instantly blame in order to deal with distressing emotions. They don't lose their temper with others or with inanimate objects, they don't smash the keyboard when the laptop messes up, they don't kick kennel doors when the dog barks for attention.

But if you have consciously chosen to go to your room and punch the pillow and scream to get something out of your system in response to your emotions, then so long as that is your choice, so long as you have taken ownership of that response and so long as responding that way does not cause you or others more distress, then so be it. That is your choice and it still shows a degree of self-regulation in that you made a conscious decision to respond in that way.

Self-regulation is not about turning off our emotions or turning our back on our emotions. In contrast, if we are acutely self-aware and totally in tune with our feelings both good and distressing, only then can we be the master of our behaviour in response. It is very empowering to be able to choose our internal response as well as our external reaction in a given situation. This can only (and yet surprisingly easily) be achieved with conscious effort.

Motivation

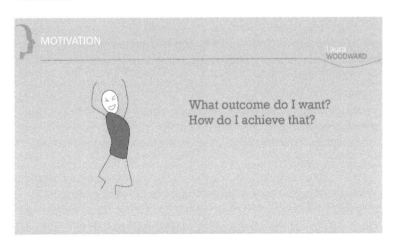

What do I want and how can I achieve it?

It's okay to want something out of a given situation. And it's okay to get what we want. Being 'responsibly selfish' means taking charge of our needs without detrimental effect to others.

For example, if a client is angry with me on the phone because I haven't done a procedure on their pet yet, probably what I want out of that situation is for the client to stop giving me a hard time and to allow me to get off the phone and to get back to doing the procedures.

That's what I want. How do I achieve that?

I stop, pause and think.

Will reflexively ranting back at the client get me what I want? Unlikely.

Will I achieve my aim by telling the client that we've had several emergencies come in which have moved their procedure down the list? Possibly.

Will using my social skills and empathy with the pet owner get me off the phone rapidly and back to doing what they and I want to be doing? Probably.

It may seem like wasting time – sitting there on the phone quietly and actively listening to them air their anxieties in angry tones at me. However, in my experience, it's the fastest way to go back to my procedures. The important thing is to pause and figure out the best outcome for you and then try to manage the situation accordingly.

I'm running late while driving somewhere. Someone cuts in front of me when I had the right of way. It's easy to be morally in the right and seething.

What do I want out of the situation and how do I achieve that?

I want to get from A to B as fast as possible. So, will tailgating this driver achieve that? Unlikely. They might drive at a snail's pace in return.

Will passing them at a dodgy turn get me what I want? Even the mildest of car bumps adds hours onto a journey.

Possibly the best way to get what I want is to not react. That's so hard, especially when they are breaking the law, but if I want to be responsibly selfish, I might choose that course of action.

Motivation takes time at first and then it becomes second nature.

Another example:

I'm receiving numerous abusive or just nasty messages from someone. What do I want out of this situation and how do I achieve that?

Possibly I want them to change their ways. How likely is wishing for that going to get me what I want? Maybe asking them will achieve it. Maybe blocking them is the only way to stop them sending the bile in my direction.

The thing is that you decide for you what you want, and then proceed in a healthy, compassionate and non-destructive way. It is possible to block someone and to be compassionate at the same time.

Empathy

Empathy has a whole chapter to itself following on directly after this one and it's one of my favourite topics. Through studying empathy, I learnt so much about human behaviour.

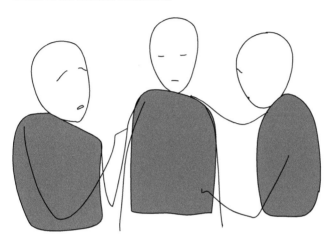

Social Skills

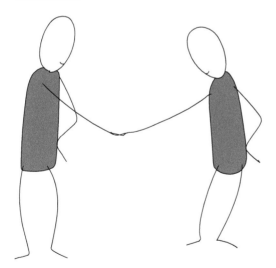

Social skills are the skills we use to communicate in an intelligent and effective way. Good eye contact, if the other person feels comfortable with it, is one component of these skills. Knowing when the other person doesn't want direct eye contact is perception, another skill.

Our body language conveys so much. For example, not standing with a consulting table between me and the pet owner shows I am listening, open to them and their concerns, approachable. Folded arms gives a signal of defensiveness.

Similarly, when with friends, having my phone out and on the coffee table says 'I'm listening to you unless something better or more important comes up'.

Eloquence can be learned. Knowing how to speak and how to listen is discussed in the next chapter on empathy.

Empathy

- The three types of empathy
- Leadership and empathy for line managers
- The evidence-based case for leadership: empathic concern versus empathy alone
- The empathy–profitability link

The Three Types of Empathy

So, empathy is one of the five components of emotional intelligence. But what is it actually? And why is it so important a quality in effective leaders?

Daniel Goleman, the father of emotional intelligence, has described three types of empathy which I feel the veterinary world cannot do without. In this climate of small practices being bought up by bigger practices who are then swallowed whole by enormous corporates, surely we need to be working harder than ever to create a sense of rapport and emotional connection amongst those on the 'shop floor'.

Cognitive Empathy

The first type of empathy is **cognitive empathy**.

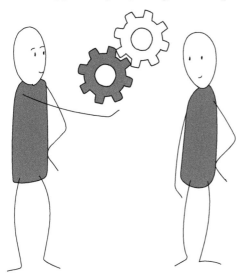

By using cognitive empathy, we can gain a better understanding of how the other person's mind works. We can see things from their perspective. We understand the language they use and can use similar language back to them effectively so that they hear us. Cognitive empathy is essential when giving performance feedback, for example. It is essential when communicating with clients. Communication is key.

However, the downside to cognitive empathy is that it can be used to manipulate others in an unkind fashion by people with twisted motivations – bullies in the workplace, for example, and narcissists.

Narcissistic Manipulation

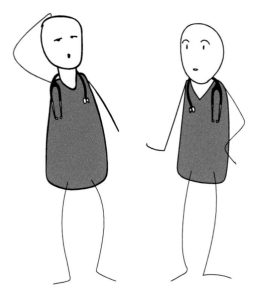

We all know someone who is emotionally abusive. They can manipulate using language and twisted methods.

Emotional Empathy

The second type of empathy, **emotional empathy**, means 'I feel with you', 'I can feel your distress'. However, I can also rejoice in your good news which brings team members together at joyful times. Narcissists typically lack this second type of empathy.

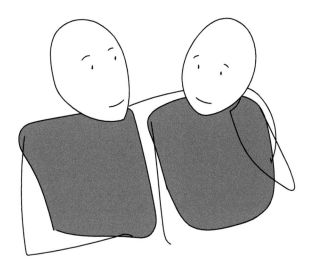

Emotional empathy is essential for good leadership, for effective team-work and for understanding the needs and desires of our clients.

When running at high levels, emotional empathy creates a sense of rapport with clients and an emotional connection between team members which gives rise to an overall harmony in the team. These teams are more productive as a result.

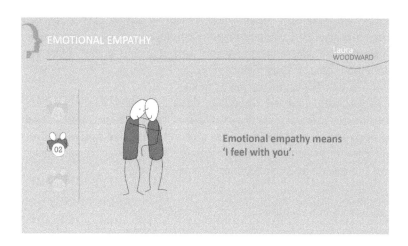

EMOTIONAL EMPATHY

Laura WOODWARD

02

Emotional empathy means 'I feel with you'.

The downside to emotional empathy is that if you are a leader who takes it upon themselves to be the sounding board for the team, without the ability to metabolise other people's concerns, it can lead to emotional exhaustion and eventually to emotional burnout.

As a counsellor in my own practice, and also as a team member in my veterinary practice to whom colleagues in distress will turn, I have to exercise a degree of self-regulation to avoid emotional burnout.

Counsellors debrief and therefore unload emotional burdens we receive from our clients onto supervisors, who in turn debrief onto other supervisors, and so the chain of avoiding emotional exhaustion and burnout is strong. However, alongside that chain of debriefing, we must use self-awareness to be conscious of the toll it takes on us, and self-regulation to avoid it burdening us and affecting our own mental wellbeing.

Also, as part of our training, we learn how to metabolise the distress we experience through counselling others.

Without formal training and supervision, it is very difficult, if not impossible, to avoid becoming distressed if you are the person to whom your colleagues and clients come when they are suffering.

Empathic Concern

The third type of empathy is **empathic concern** – 'When I see that you are in distress, I have an overwhelming need to help you out'.

These are the proactive leaders who speak to the Veterinary Defence Society on their vet's behalf when something terrible has happened. They organise the CPD for struggling employees. They see someone is distressed and take them somewhere for a confidential chat before the situation escalates. They fund counselling for team members who need it *before* the crisis or resignation happens.

In successful practices, especially these days when many of us are working for corporate practices, these three types of empathy need to be running at full capacity from grass roots up to HR and well beyond in order for those facing the customers to thrive, be productive and proactive and remain in the professions for their working life.

Leadership and Empathy for Line Managers

The greatest leaders allow others to thrive based on their strengths.

How to Use Empathy to Enhance Your Leadership Status

> *A manager's leadership style is responsible for 30% of the business's profitability.*
>
> Daniel Goleman in Harvard Business Review, April 2000

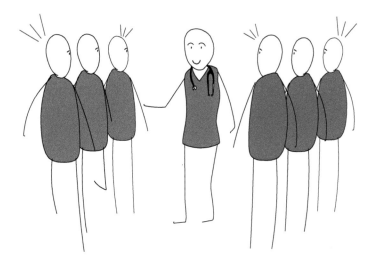

Daniel Goleman did some work in the States drawing on research involving over 3000 executives, published in 'Leadership That Gets Results' (https://hbr.org/2000/03/leadership-that-gets-results). The research concludes that a manager's leadership style was responsible for 30% of the business's profitability; that isn't just money but staff productivity and engagement, creating a negative or positive 'working atmosphere'.

Empathy can result in greater profitability in our practices. How can I, as a leader, show by example how cognitive empathy, emotional empathy and empathic concern can become part of who we are as individuals, leading to greater success at work?

Cognitive empathy means I understand how to listen to the team as a whole and I can communicate with individual team members by listening, understanding and feeding back.

That's the upside. The downside is that communication has to be tailored to the individual and varying needs of the team members, requiring more one-to-one meetings as well as group staff meetings. It's time-consuming.

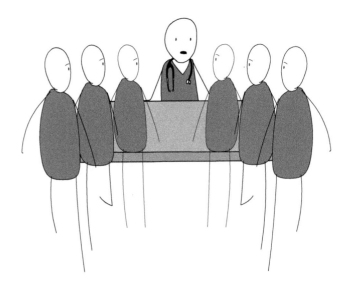

Emotional empathy creates a leader who can assess staff morale as it changes from day to day. If management has emotional empathy running at high levels, it creates a rapport amongst the team and decreases the communication gap between management and staff. However, it requires flexibility and the ability to change tack at short notice. Leadership can and should be situational, depending on the needs of the team.

Empathically concerned leaders create highly bonded teams. These are the leaders who organise CPD for vets who are struggling clinically, the line managers who remember if a nurse's parent has cancer and makes sure they have compassionate leave, the head vet who knows the name of every receptionist and patient care assistant (PCA), the manager who books mental wellbeing seminars for the team that's lost direction.

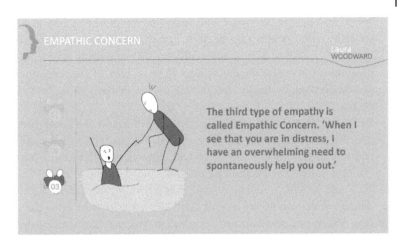

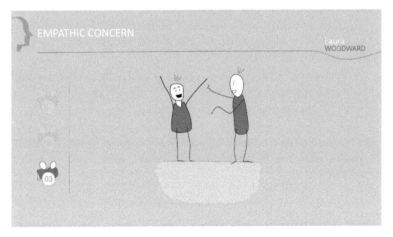

So how do I cultivate authentic empathy at all three levels in myself so that it becomes part of the culture of the team? How do I learn the difference between empathy, sympathy and apathy and their impact on the human connection?

- *Mindfulness mini-meditations*: spend 20 minutes each morning clearing your mind and attaining pinpoint concentration on your breathing. Then consciously decide to make the effort, one day at a time, to be more mindful of hidden cues in others, and to understand the 'emotional data' in your staff. This increases cognitive and emotional empathy. It takes effort at the start and then becomes a habit and eventually it will be a firm personality trait. Then putting your 'compassionate hat' on for the day, resolve to be mindful of your thoughts and actions at work, i.e. be acutely aware of each thought and each action.

- *Make yourself aware* of how lack of empathy in one-to-one encounters has the potential to abolish any positive effects which that time-consuming encounter could have had, hinders communication and can even cause psychological harm.
- *Resolve to be more emotionally intelligent* where you can. Identify and manage your own emotions and those of your staff more effectively, thus setting the standard for behaviour in the practice. Understand yourself better to safeguard your own mental health and personal wellbeing. Be more reflective personally and professionally, thus having empathy but not becoming emotionally exhausted with sympathy.
- *Listen more actively*: pause to digest and absorb what has been conveyed to you.
- *Understand reflective leadership* and how to use these skills for staff wellbeing and productivity. Respond with wisdom and show that you have tailored your response to the individual.

> *Between stimulus and response there is a space. In that space is our power to choose our response. In our response lies our growth and our freedom.*
>
> Viktor E. Frankl

- *Plan one act of empathic concern* each day at work, thus avoiding apathy and showing the team that you are a leader who is not jaded.

Empathy breeds empathy. By showing you have a high emotional quotient (EQ) as well as a high IQ, your charisma and leadership status improve in the eyes of your team. It becomes infectious. Don't be bashful about it. Spell it out and be honest.

> *Leaders influence the team's mood. The team's mood drives performance. What's your conclusion?*
>
> Joshua Freedman, CEO of Six Seconds Emotional Intelligence Training

The Evidence-based Case for Leadership: Empathic Concern versus Empathy Alone

In January 2022, in the Potential Project's Human Leader Study, a biannual study of 5000 companies across 100 countries, leaders were asked if they were more likely to be in the empathy class or the empathic concern class. The results were then correlated with both the leaders' and employees' experiences at work.

The study showed that leaders who rate themselves high on empathic concern report 63% lower burnout, 66% lower stress levels and a staggering 200% lower intent to quit their organisation compared to leaders who rated themselves in the empathy only group. They felt more confidence in their ability to lead others and were less likely to experience personal distress or be overwhelmed by negative emotions.

More specifically, the data show that leaders with a less proactive empathy preference have a 12% increased risk of burnout on average compared to their more proactive empathic concern counterparts.

> To put this into perspective, a 12% increase in risk for burnout translates directly into an 11% increase in mortality risk for leaders.

The picture is similarly positive for employees being led by proactive leaders; they are 25% more engaged in their jobs and 20% more committed to the organisation. Not surprisingly, they too have an 11% lower risk of burnout.

Acceptance and Proactivity

As mindfulness teachers, we often teach our clients to sit with difficult emotions. To name them, look them in the eye and accept them, versus avoidance which is often our normal reactive response.

That doesn't mean we can't also take steps to alleviate the difficulties.

Pain is inevitable – suffering is optional. Although life's difficulties are often beyond our control, suffering is to a large extent determined by how we react to these difficulties. Our reaction can be under our control. Such is the power of the mind.

We can spend an hour sitting on the cushion deciding our emotional reaction to a given stimulus. We can also spend time being proactive about tackling difficult situations. It's not contrary to the teaching of mindfulness. It's a true human reaction.

When leaders and team members go the extra mile for others, the team becomes visibly and tangibly stronger and more intact.

Empathy is when we see someone suffer, understand the suffering they experience and sit together with them. This is a good, altruistic response but *empathic concern* is different. Empathic concern involves taking a step back from empathy and asking ourselves 'What can I do to proactively support the person who is suffering?' while empathising with them at the same time.

How Do I Do It?

Wouldn't it be great if our members were able to take care of their own mental wellbeing? If only we could hand that responsibility onto them, with our support of course, it would free up so much time for us as leaders. That would be proactive empathic concern.

As psychotherapeutic counsellors, we know that if a client designs their own wellbeing programme and meditation techniques, it is so much more valid than if it were all determined by us the therapists.

Being aware of the impact of the practice on each member of the team is a start. It's surprisingly difficult and time-consuming to do this. The building, the IT issues, the structure of breaks, the volume of the phones all matter.

What's Not Helpful

- Putting a poster on the toilet door with various numbers to phone if you're in crisis is very common. It's rarely helpful although it does tick a box on the list of health and safety requirements as an employer. It's done with good intentions.
- The reality is that once your employee is in crisis, they don't have the will or energy to make these phone calls. And even if they did, the waiting lists are months long.
- You can plaster helpline adverts and posters the length of the most populated corridor in the practice. I know, because I have counselled hundreds of vets and nurses, that something different needs to be done.
- Webinars on how to look after your mental health are superb. If your staff logged on. But they don't. I ask many of my patients why they don't log on. It's because the last thing they want to do after work is to log back on to work.

The proof?

In the Mind Matters Initiative (MMI) survey 2021, 70% of respondents had personally experienced a mental health concern, yet only half had received professional support; 75% said they knew where to access mental health support if they needed it.

What Is Helpful

- True empathic concern combined with proactive leadership means that the leader will organise seminars for the staff which they attend in real time during work hours. The consultations are blanked out for the day, the venue is close to work or in the practice itself, the phones are turned off, lunch is provided.
- The seminar is not about how to make a consultation into a profitable procedure this time. It's teaching your staff how to take care of their own mental wellbeing so that they don't need the phone numbers on the back of the toilet door.
- It's about training them in techniques and giving them the tools to deal with crises and pandemics and life's ups and downs.
- This will also free up time for the leaders to concentrate on other matters if their workforce now has the tools to look after their own mental health. It's a win–win.

> Happiness comes through our deeper humanistic experiences like doing purposeful work, caring for others, being generous and making authentic connections. Isn't this the description of being a vet and a vet nurse?

Happiness is the long-term state of experiencing a meaningful, purposeful and positive life. Being a veterinary professional is meaningful, purposeful and can be the most positive of vocations if we have the knowledge of how to see and feel these experiences.

Empathic concern from leaders positively impacts organisational commitment, job performance and engagement, and decreases the incidence of burnout.

When leaders approach difficult situations with empathic concern, they help to encourage genuine human interactions, lifting not just the business but our inter-staff relationships and our people, too.

Source: Some of the above text is adapted from *Compassionate Leadership: How to Do Hard Things in Human Way* by Rasmus Hougaard and Jacqueline Carter, published by Harvard Business Review Press, January 18, 2022.

The Empathy–Profitability Link

The truly empathic vet and nurse can directly increase profitability on a daily basis.

So very briefly to recap, the first type of empathy is cognitive empathy and this basically means that I understand the way your mind works and I understand the language you use. I can communicate with you, reflecting back to you with the language you understand, and I can show you that I understand you.

The second type of empathy is emotional empathy – 'I feel with you'. In other words, I can sense when you are happy, distressed, stressed or concerned, whether you have expressed those thoughts out loud or not.

The third and most powerful kind of empathy is empathic concern. This means that when I see that you are distressed, I have an overwhelming need to help you out. I need to make your life easier, and I can.

As vets and nurses on the front line of customer care, we need to have all three kinds of empathy running at high levels if we are to offer the best service to our clients and the best care to their pets. Increased profitability naturally follows on from this.

Cognitive empathy training improves our communication skills with clients and each other. I can actively listen to the client, they feel listened to and understood. I can ask the right questions in a way that puts the client at ease and gets me the history I need. The client trusts me because they know that I can hear what they are saying. When I suggest options for diagnosis and treatment, because I am on their wavelength, they are more likely to proceed because of that trust.

When I discuss the client and their pet at handovers, hospital rounds, referrals, etc., I have an exact picture of their requirements. But, more importantly, because I can also understand the way my colleagues communicate and the way that their individual minds work, we all can understand what the client wants and I can hand this case over to my colleagues with confidence, knowing that communication is excellent.

Emotional empathy, when running at high levels, enables me to see beyond the words that can be so hastily spoken in the consulting room, especially when stress levels are running high. I can see and feel the emotions of the client and of their pet.

By sensing emotions and putting them into words for the client ('I imagine you're worried about the anaesthetic'), we create a rapport with them which further strengthens their trust and faith in us.

The body language of a pet owner can speak volumes about their fears, money concerns, sadness and even distrust. The vet and nurse with good emotional empathy can interpret body language and put it into words for the client. Profit-wise, the nervous client may be reassured by more detailed preanaesthetic tests. The anxious client may feel less anxious if we are more indepth with our investigations. The stressed client may want their pet hospitalised rather than observed at home. If we offer, the client may take us up on it and be pleased that we thought to see beyond their words and 'read their mind'. If they don't take us up on what we offer, they are likely to feel the same degree of trust and relief that we felt their distress and offered what was appropriate to them at that time as opposed to a bunch of 'extras' for the hell of it.

> Offering in the right way, at the right time, shows good rapport rather than a thirst for commission.

Emotional empathy within a team creates strong bonds. We celebrate each other's joy and offer support in times of need. We can feel when our colleague is swamped and doesn't want to get involved in another case. Similarly, we can identify the team member who is eager to get involved and take the case forward appropriately.

Empathic concern is the type of empathy which we would wish all vets and nurses to have as a natural strong personality trait. Empathic concern is the kind of empathy which earns us five-star Google reviews, boxes of chocolate and fully paid bills. And it is the type of empathy which makes us truly compassionate people who gain pleasure each day from our work despite the many events which could turn our mood in the other direction.

'I feel your distress and I have an overwhelming need to help you out'. This is the vet who sees that the owner needs us to keep their pet overnight and offers it before the client has even realised it's an option.

This is the nurse who senses the terror in their client and bumps their pet up to the top of the ops list, thus reducing their hours of anxious waiting to a minimum.

This is the vet who makes it a matter of urgency to phone the client as soon as their pet is recovered from their general anaesthetic and if there is no answer, sends a reassuring text.

It's the nurse who phones the day after a procedure to see how the pet and client are, and the PCA who takes the time to get to know the pet and lets the owner know that we are aware that their pet likes ear scratches, neck massage, squeaky toys, and gravy instead of jelly.

Secular Buddhist Concepts

- Basic elements of secular Buddhism
- The Four Noble Truths
- The nature of impermanence
- Attachment
- Positive psychology
- The three circles of control

> Do not try to use what you learn from Buddhism to be a better Buddhist; use it to be a better whatever-you-already-are.

Basic Elements of Secular Buddhism

Secular Buddhists share a sceptical view of the supernatural deities and processes of traditional Buddhism such as rebirth, etc. However, they use traditional Buddhist concepts to develop a more mindful and compassionate life.

Secular and non-secular Buddhists can have fantastic debates on metaphysics and deities, as I often have with my mentor, a Sri Lankan Buddhist monk. Compassion and humour are abundant.

For secular Buddhists, the Buddha is seen as an historical person, not a deity. We approach the Dharma as ethical dimensions of Buddhism to guide us rather than as a set of religious beliefs.

Secular Buddhists try to create a society which promotes the flourishing of all, as well as transforming ourselves to achieve true happiness.

The Four Noble Truths

The teachings of the Buddha are condensed in the Four Noble Truths and the Eightfold Path. Interpreted into lay language, it makes for interesting and intellectually stimulating reading.

> *For fast-acting relief, try slowing down.*
>
> Lily Tomlin

Mental Wellbeing and Positive Psychology for Veterinary Professionals: A Pre-emptive, Proactive and Solution-based Approach, First Edition. Laura Woodward.
© 2024 John Wiley & Sons Ltd. Published 2024 by John Wiley & Sons Ltd.

'I teach suffering, its origin, cessation and path. That's all I teach', declared the Buddha 2500 years ago.

So, in lay person's terms, what is it all about and how does Buddhism teach calm and joy? My understanding is this.

The Truth of Suffering

It may sound a bit miserable and pessimistic, but suffering is all around us. Bear with me. Apart from the obvious hardships of old age, sickness and death, life is full of unfulfilled plans, shattered dreams and yearning for things to be better. Seriously, don't stop reading just yet.

The Truth of the Origin of Suffering

The Buddha taught that basically, the reason we suffer is because of desire or a yearning for things to be different. This is broken down into *Greed*: we want more of what we think will make us happy; *Delusion*: we are ignorant when it comes to what will actually bring us happiness; and *Hatred*: a rather hyperbolic term for being unkind to others.

The Cessation of Suffering

At last, some good news: the Buddha taught that the way to extinguish desire, which causes suffering, is to liberate oneself from attachment – liberation from the constant yearning for things to be different and for things to happen which we believe will help us to finally reach our 'goal' of happiness.

We often feel that once this goal is reached or that event happens, we will finally be happy. Once I have that dream job, it will be okay. Once I have x number of kids, I will feel complete. So long as there's great snow on that skiing holiday, it will be a good holiday and we'll all live happily ever after.

If we can let go of our attachment to these ideals and instead allow the ups and downs of life to happen non-judgementally, life really does become far less disappointing. Once those disappointments are gone, it's easier to appreciate the many tiny, good things which previously went unnoticed.

> If things are tough, just notice the sadness. It won't last.
> If things are rosy, notice the joy. It won't last.

Everything changes, nothing stays the same and that's okay. Learning to accept the *impermanence* of everything helps us to ride the ups and downs without the need to judge every event as 'good' or 'bad'. It stops us desperately trying to hold onto a good moment as it fades into the past. It prevents us from killing time until the holiday arrives so that we realise that we can enjoy our time now as well as our time then.

The Path to the Cessation of Suffering

So how do we do it? Achieving Nirvana and everything along the way.

Well, the Eightfold Path is not something to be undertaken lightly. There are no shortcuts and, to be honest, we are unlikely to reach full enlightenment or Nirvana. But the reason behind at least being educated in the Path is that knowing about it leads to enough emotional nourishment to encourage even the busiest of us to give it a shot. And, in giving it a shot, the effects are immediately noticeable. Otherwise, how else would mindfulness have achieved so much acclaim?

The eight stages are not to be taken in order, but rather support and reinforce each other.

1) *Right Understanding* – accepting Buddhist teachings. Basically, reading this synopsis and deciding if it can guide you.
2) *Right Intention* – a commitment to cultivate the right attitudes.
3) *Right Speech* – speaking truthfully, avoiding slander, gossip and abusive speech. This can be hard to do.
4) *Right Action* – behaving peacefully and harmoniously.
5) *Right Livelihood* – avoiding making a living in ways that cause harm, such as exploiting people, drug dealing, etc. Hopefully, for most of us, this is relatively easy to do.
6) *Right Effort* – cultivating positive states of mind. This doesn't just happen because we yearn for it. We have to put in the effort and the hours. For many of us, that means an hour less sleep every night so we can meditate pre-dawn. For others, it means making a conscious effort to spend 10 minutes every day in mini-meditation.
7) *Right Mindfulness* – developing awareness of the body, sensations, feelings and states of mind. Meditating and self-awareness.
8) *Right Concentration* – developing the mental focus necessary for this awareness. Meditation takes practice; it gets easier each time you do it.

The eight stages can be grouped into Wisdom (right understanding and intention), Ethical Conduct (right speech, action and livelihood) and Meditation (right effort, mindfulness and concentration).

The Buddha described the Eightfold Path as a means to enlightenment, like a raft for crossing a river. Once one has reached the opposite shore, one no longer needs the raft and can leave it behind.

> The vast majority of us will never reach the opposite shore. But the gentle cruising on the river is worth the effort it takes to get onto the raft.

The Nature of Impermanence

Attachment to possessions and achievement invariably leads to disappointment and disillusionment because everything is impermanent.

Everything changes, nothing stays the same and that can be okay.

> *Nothing is permanent – not even our troubles.*
>
> Charlie Chaplin

Impermanence is constant change and it's woven into the very fabric of our existence. Moments come and they go. Years go by. Kids grow up too fast. Holidays take ages to arrive and seemingly minutes to pass. Time flies when you're having fun. The breath you took five minutes ago is long gone.

Intellectually, we understand that our pet will be born, age and die, that our car will break down, that the traffic jam will eventually move. Our work is to move that understanding from our intellect and nestle it deep in our hearts. But how does that benefit us? Sounds miserable, right?

There's a beauty to impermanence. In Japan, people flock to see the spring blossoming of the cherry trees. The festival is over after a few days, as are the blooms. Tiny blue flax flowers in North America last for just a day. Glastonbury is amazing. But it has to end because it's impossible to party that hard for longer than three or four days.

Impermanence isn't a good or a bad thing. It's just a fact. We rely on constant change; we rely on impermanence.

Ancient trees will burn in great forests so new ones can be born. Evil dictatorships crumble.

Winter days can be cold, wet and dark. Some people love winter. Others prefer sunshine, long warm evenings and swimming in the sea. How many winters have you seen pass and give way to spring and summer? We need winters to be impermanent.

So how does really understanding impermanence benefit our wellbeing? If you're having a great day, enjoy it to its fullest, it won't last.

And if your day is feeling like a disaster, hang in there, it won't last.

No matter how long that ops list is, it will eventually all get done. That's also the nature of impermanence.

If you're dreading the root canal treatment you're having next week, have faith that that day will come. And it will go. And the root canal procedure will be done.

So, how can I claim that impermanence is a path to fulfilment and an antidote to regret? Accepting the nature of impermanence is a key Buddhist teaching. It also leads neatly into relinquishing attachments which, according to Buddhist teachings, are one cause of suffering.

Impermanence Versus Attachment

So, if I can accept that I am impermanent, as is my cat, my job, this good or bad day, my holiday, then I can hold myself back from becoming so *attached* to the necessity of it being permanent that I can relax a little. Instead of fearing and dreading the end of my holiday, I can enjoy it even more mindfully and embrace every tiny joyous thing about it even though I know that it will pass.

With time, I can accept that everything, even all humans on earth, including me, is fleeting in some way. That is acceptance and letting go of my attachment and desperate need. And that's okay.

Attachment

According to Buddhism, attachment is the root of suffering, and it is usually the reason why impermanence is difficult to fathom for many people. Rationally accepting that everyone and everything is temporary is a refreshing and at the same time daunting concept, and whether you want to believe it or not, it's true.

Positive Psychology

While clinical psychology has largely focused on diagnosing and treating mental illness and diseases, positive psychology is concerned with cultivating positive wellbeing, which is *very* different from merely eliminating negative mental states.

We already know that external factors don't determine our happiness. Certainly, positive external factors compound and complement our overall contentment, but internal factors are required to achieve an authentically joyous life. True happiness comes from within.

So, although a fortnight in the Maldives would be fantastic right now, it would come and then it would be over, i.e. it is impermanent. Then you are still the same person (although a bit more rested), left with your mental state which only you can cultivate.

It is also important to understand that grasping for positive thoughts, emotions and occurrences in life is not what positive psychology suggests. If you accept the notion of impermanence but still attempt to constantly force happiness and joy into your life, you are missing the point.

This quote from Paul T.P. Wong (2007), a positive psychologist, sums up the concept of impermanence and attachment:

> *Craving for happiness necessarily causes us to fear or reject anything that causes unhappiness or pain.*
>
> *Attachment to possession and achievement invariably leads to disappointment and disillusionment because everything is impermanent.*
>
> *Thus, the positive psychology of pursuing positive experiences and avoiding negative experiences is counterproductive, because the very focus on happiness contains the seed of unhappiness and suffering. Failure to embrace life's experience in its entirety is at the root of suffering.*

The Three Circles of Control

So much has been written about the mental health impact of the three circles of control. You know that when you try not to feel something like anxiety or sadness, it just comes back bigger and stronger. Even if we assume a zombie-like, emotionless mode through alcohol or drugs or even just binge watching Netflix, once the numbness wears off, it still hurts and sometimes it hurts even more because we haven't accepted any of the pain.

As one example, the war in Ukraine is different on so many levels, coming so soon after the global COVID-19 pandemic. For one thing, this time there is a perpetrator. While our minds have to deal with familiar emotions like anxiety, fear and despair, we now have anger to add to the mix. Helplessness, hopelessness and guilt are in there too.

In counselling psychology, there is a concept called the *circles of control* which helps us to understand and reflect on whether things that affect us are amenable to our personal influence. The idea here is that some things – many things, in fact – happen that are entirely beyond your influence, so your energy is better focused on things that you can influence.

In the *central circle* are things that we can control. Although it may take effort and instruction, we can make changes here for the better. This includes the most important thing of all: our mind. With good instruction, we can literally change our minds. Mindfulness can rapidly move our chaotic way of thinking and reflexive way of behaving into an easy and methodical way of thinking and a way of behaving which is reflective rather than reflexive, i.e. we decide our reactions to things.

The *middle circle* contains things over which we have a small amount of control. This will include many things: our friends, family, jobs, habits, daily life. Through compassion, self-compassion, kindness and purposeful actions, we can have an enormous beneficial effect on the people around us. Sometimes just giving off good vibes can be palpably calming for those around us. Other times, a change in our daily habits can turn our profound sadness into joy. I say this from personal experience of horrific tragedy and soon afterwards feeling blissful about tiny things around me.

The *outer circle* is made up of things we cannot control. Vladimir Putin is going to pursue his military agenda whatever you or I think, do or say, so this sits in our outer circle, beyond any kind of control we might have.

So, how can we just accept it? We see the Ukrainian people resist and fight back with unfathomable resilience and bravery. The public awareness is phenomenal thanks to President Zelensky keeping Ukraine in the forefront of the minds of everyone around the globe. We're angry and want to see Putin accountable.

Acceptance is not about sitting there like a blancmange doing nothing and saying 'Que sera, sera'. It's not about being complacent and ineffectual.

Acceptance is about feeling that anger and maybe pure unadulterated hatred for the perpetrators of human tragedy and accepting that we feel that way.

So, we can have all that anger within us, for obvious reasons, and still be kind to those in our inner circle (ourselves) and our middle circle.

We can donate cash, we can drive a truckload of blankets to Poland, all the time allowing ourselves to feel anger, grief and the excitement that comes with being proactive all at the same time.

The Serenity Prayer was written in the 1800s by Reinhold Neibuhr (1892–1971). Its popularity grew in the 1940s when Alcoholics Anonymous started using a shortened version for its recovery programme.

> *God grant me the serenity*
> *To accept the things I cannot change.*
> *Courage to change the things I can.*
> *And wisdom to know the difference.*
> *Living one day at a time.*
> *Enjoying one moment at a time.*

By accepting our plethora of emotions one by one, maybe we will actually be more effective and courageous in the long run in changing the things we can and being wise to the things we can't.

Reference

Wong, P. T.P. (2007). Chinese Positive Psychology. International Network on Personal Meaning. www.meaning.ca/archives/archive/art_Chinese-PP_P_ Wong.htm

Part 2

How to Meditate

Mindful meditation doesn't change life. Life remains as fragile and as unpredictable as ever.

How to Meditate: Part 1

- Introduction
- Gain control of your mind
- Mindful drinking
- Mindful breathing
- Mindful body scan
- Loving kindness meditation
- Hand-on-heart meditation

> Most people can equate the number of minutes they spend concentrating on 'nothingness' with their level of calmness, and often happiness, that very day.

Introduction

During mindful meditation, we get inside our own head, we calm it down and create a safe, open space. Once there, we can do anything we want within that clear space.

It may be that this time, we choose to look at our emotions one at a time. It's important to not 'become' an emotion but rather to observe it as an onlooker with a curious, non-judgemental mindset.

Once identified, it can be so much easier to choose our response to that emotion. Once decided, that response becomes what happens next, simply because we have chosen it.

During other meditations, maybe we want to explore something else. For example, maybe I'm feeling anxious and I do or don't know why. During that meditation, I can explore the anxiety and see if there's a reason for it which I can see. Maybe I then choose what to do next, or to not change anything. Often, just figuring out why I have a knot in my stomach is enough to ease the discomfort.

We can use imagery, talking to an empty chair, letting go, anything we choose. Often, prior to meditation, I will have decided what I want out of

Mental Wellbeing and Positive Psychology for Veterinary Professionals: A Pre-emptive, Proactive and Solution-based Approach, First Edition. Laura Woodward.
© 2024 John Wiley & Sons Ltd. Published 2024 by John Wiley & Sons Ltd.

that session. For me, that might help. Other times, I can just be present with a calm, clear mind for as long as I choose.

For very basic meditation, step by step we are aiming to:

- gain control of our busy mind (simply explained, but not easy)
- learn how to clear a space within our mind
- practise staying there.

So many people tell me 'I don't have time to meditate'. That is so understandable in a world where we're multitasking from waking to sleeping.

Others say they get everything they need from playing tennis for an hour, swimming, running, etc. For that hour, we are so caught up in what we're doing that it feels as though we are hopping off the world for 60 minutes for a breather. And it feels good. It can be looked on as a form of mindfulness: focusing our minds on the present moment, on purpose.

Distraction from all that's going in our heads and in our lives is nearly always welcomed as a break. And that's part of the reason we become hooked on tennis/soap operas/books/watching sport.

Others argue that, if we took the time to meditate and to identify (but not to OVER identify) with all that's going on in our head, then the tennis, run, etc. would become even more enjoyable, as it wouldn't be under pressure to be the only means by which we grab an hour of sanity. In other words, if we can observe and accept our emotions during meditation, we no longer feel the need to escape from them.

So mindful meditation can't be a bad thing, it's just a question of when to fit it in. It isn't easy at all but it is very simple. It takes practice. The first few times, you may be distracted after five seconds. With daily practice, you can achieve up to an hour or more of meaningful meditation, with instant results.

During counselling, I often teach my clients how to do the most basic of meditations: meditation on the breath or a simple body scan meditation.

I have never met anyone who didn't feel good after a 10-minute basic meditation.

We can try it out for 10 minutes each morning for three days. How achievable is that? Even after such a small dip of your toes into these unknown waters, the effects will be felt and you can decide if you want to take it further or not. There is no right or wrong answer.

> On morning meditations, once is a start, twice and you've set a precedent. Three times and it's become your new normal. The goal is to explore morning meditations, not to become a monk by next month.

So, to start, let's focus on gaining control of our mind and emptying it of junk. Anyone can learn to meditate. I urge you to do this every morning so that it becomes a habit, a way of life.

With very little time, you will become masterful at this and be ready for another step: learning how to observe and deal with one emotion at a time, and formulate your internal and external responses to those emotions.

A useful challenge would be to set aside half an hour each morning to practise. Having a coffee while you get settled makes it less torturous. How do you do this? You could leave your normal morning alarm as it is, then make a second alarm for 30 minutes earlier. That way you have literally 'created time' for your practice.

It's so important to just switch off the alarm and not quickly scroll through your phone. That can all wait until your normal alarm rings, if that's how you want to start the day. You don't have to worry about being so 'in the zone' that you forget to start the day. After 30 minutes, you'll be rudely reminded to do just that.

So, coffee in hand, find a comfortable place to sit alone – on your bed, on a cushion on the floor or on the sofa, etc., away from your people and your pets. We aim to be alert, so sit upright, legs crossed or not.

Gain Control of Your Mind

Easier said than done. Mornings are often the time of day when we are frantically triaging all that needs to be done. Remember you've got up early to do this, you have 'made time'. So the day's organising can wait until you are finished. Methods to gain control can include mindful coffee drinking, mindful breathing and body scan exercises. It can actually be fun, it doesn't have to be deadly serious.

Mindful Drinking

So, look at the coffee and concentrate on it. Feel the heat of the cup on each hand. Smell the coffee. Feel the temperature as you take a drink. Taste it in every part of your mouth. Observe it being swallowed. Listen to your swallowing sounds. Taste the aftertaste. See if you can feel a caffeine hit with each sip.

If you have concentrated on mindful drinking and nothing else for one minute, you are doing well. Over the month, a good aim would be to extend this time to five minutes.

Each time you find yourself going off on a tangent, don't berate yourself, it's not a mistake. Just gently come back to the present moment and the task in hand.

Mindful Breathing

Now try to just sit and observe your breathing. It doesn't have to be active deep breaths, just notice the fact that you are breathing and focus on the tip of your nose or on the space between your eyes (sometimes we call this the 'third eye').

If this is difficult, try counting your breaths. See if you can get to 60 without your mind wandering away. If it does, gently bring your focus back. Maybe for the first few sessions you can only get to five breaths before your mind wanders off. Remember that every time you extend your pinpoint concentration by one breath, you are becoming more masterful at meditation.

Mindful Body Scan

So now you're awake, mindful body scan is another great way to be mindful. Focusing on 'nothing' is extremely hard to do for lengthy periods of time. Beginners find it easier to focus on something. Body scan involves total concentration on individual parts of our body one at a time from your toes to the top of your head, gradually moving up along your body. The slower you can do it without losing focus, the greater will be the benefits. If you are managing to concentrate well, slow it down further.

With your eyes open or closed (as most people prefer), and having cleared your mind with a breath meditation for however long you chose, focus on one of your feet.

Try not to move or wriggle the parts you're focusing on, just notice their position, temperature, whether they ache, itch, etc.

If you find an ache or an itch, try to observe it without moving or scratching. I'll explain later.

Slowly, very slowly move up to focus on your knee. Observe how it feels, then your hip, then your seat.

Do the same with the other foot to seat.

Move your focus slowly up your back, to your shoulders (usually plenty of tension to notice there), along the back of your scalp to the top of your head.

Then focus on one hand, noticing each finger without moving them, one by one.

Then slowly up to your wrist, elbow and shoulder.

Do the same with your other hand to shoulder.

Starting with your pelvis, move slowly up your abdomen. Notice your posture without changing it.

Observe your abdomen and chest rise and fall with your breath, up along your neck to your jaw (often tense or clenched), your face (again rarely without tension), notice the position of your tongue, your eyes, forehead and finally up to the top of your head.

Return to observing the breath and slowly open your eyes.

One reason for not altering your position when you observe discomfort and for not scratching an itch is to practise, in a very easy and basic way, the art of acceptance. We will discuss acceptance later throughout this book and in Part Four on Acceptance and Commitment Therapy (ACT).

If you can learn to just let that itch be, it will become something you don't even notice. If you allow a bit of discomfort to be present, you will become used to that too and just accept it. It's something to play around with as you see fit.

Loving Kindness Meditation

This may sound very hippie but it's worth exploring because it's very powerful.

Again, having cleared your mind using the breath meditation or body scan or both, picture someone who is very, very dear to you and whom you love. It might be a person or an animal but for this example, I'll refer to them as a person.

Feel the emotions running between you and this person. Observe how much you love them and wish them to be happy.

There is a typical Buddhist mantra used at this stage where you imagine yourself saying to this person: 'May you be well, may you be happy, may you be peaceful'. Say it several times.

Then, imagine them saying this mantra to you. Observe any emotions you feel as you see that they love you: 'May you be well, may you be happy, may you be peaceful'.

Moving onto yourself, allow yourself to wish these good things for you: 'May I be well, may I be happy, may I be peaceful'. See if you can really mean it.

Next, imagine a group of your close friends. It doesn't matter if there are two or 20. Just bunch them together: 'May you be well, may you be happy, may you be peaceful'.

Now it gets a bit harder. Imagine a person or people who you would not normally wish good things for: 'May you be well, may you be happy, may you be peaceful'. There's no danger that this will do anything to or for these people. But it can be quite interesting to see the effect it has on you.

Now, extending this loving kindness to all the random people you'll come across that day, including everyone on the bus, the roads, the tube, at work, etc.: 'May you be well, may you be happy, may you be peaceful'.

Observe how you feel now, take a few mindful breaths and open your eyes.

I use this one a lot when driving. It can completely change your day to use it when you're in the car, bus or train. Remember that everyone around you is exactly like you and you all have a common goal: to get from A to B. So these random crowds aren't the enemy.

Try, in your head, when you see any pedestrians to say: 'May you be well, may you be happy, may you be peaceful'. Try wishing the driver in front of you the same and hope they have a good day. If someone acts like they own the road, try: 'May you be well, may you be happy, may you be peaceful'.

And to all the commuters on the train, tube and bus: 'May you be well, may you be happy, may you be peaceful'.

Hand-on-Heart Meditation

This is a very effective meditation which can bring comfort and ease sadness and anxiety through touch.

We know that oxytocin release helps us to feel nurtured and eases fear. Self-harming, where people cut their skin often with a blade or needle, releases surges of oxytocin which is one of the reasons it is so effective in providing a rush of calm. Other, non-harmful methods of releasing oxytocin include massage, foot rubs, hugging, scalp scratching, etc.

Although this is called hand-on-heart meditation because typically we place our own hand on our own heart, you can do anything you like to self-soothe using touch to provide warmth and care during this meditation.

Maybe place one or both hands on your cheeks. Or you can cradle your face in your hands. One client of mine holds her hands warmly together and rests this hand-hold on her lap. You could try hugging yourself, stroking your own face, etc. It's totally up to you.

The following description assumes you have your hand on your heart, so please adapt it to whatever you've chosen.

With your eyes closed and having cleared your mind using the breath meditation or body scan, place your hand on the centre of your chest. Feel the rise and fall of your chest as you breathe.

If you can, feel your heartbeat and realise the here and now of this meditation. Be present in this moment as intensely as you can.

Feel the increased warmth on the palm of your hand and the warmth that your hand brings to your heart.

Some people use a mantra of 'Here' as they breathe inwards and 'and now' as they breathe out to keep them focused. Others like the mantra 'It's okay. I'm okay'.

In therapy, I tailor this to each individual person. You can say whatever you please to make it personal to you.

This meditation can be used any time, anywhere for however long you choose.

> Hand-on-heart meditation is soothing and comforting whilst being empowering and liberating at the same time.

In the next section, we'll talk about how to observe an emotion without overidentifying with it, and how to formulate a plan of action when faced with that emotion.

However, it would be wise to become proficient with these first few meditations before moving onto the next practices.

How to Meditate: Part 2

- Observe an emotion
- Anger
- Anxiety

> *The greatest weapon against stress is our ability to choose one thought over another.*
>
> William James

Observe an Emotion

Now you are ready to identify one emotion you are feeling. It may be something as narrow as anger at someone for something they have done or as broad as generalised anxiety.

Conversely, it might be as broad as generalised anger or as narrow as anxiety about an impending or possible future event.

It may be an uplifting emotion of happiness, freedom or excitement. These emotions are often discarded all too rapidly by us and moved down the triage list as not needing attention because they aren't causing us distress. Ironically, embracing these emotions and identifying with them can give us the fuel needed to address the distressing emotions.

Let's observe a couple of common emotions you'll come across during these exercises. Although anger and anxiety are dealt with in more detail in Part Three, they are great examples to use when we are visualising an emotion during meditation.

Anger

Very few people celebrate feeling angry no matter how justified that anger is.

Are you enjoying the feelings of anger? Or are they disturbing?

Mental Wellbeing and Positive Psychology for Veterinary Professionals: A Pre-emptive, Proactive and Solution-based Approach, First Edition. Laura Woodward.
© 2024 John Wiley & Sons Ltd. Published 2024 by John Wiley & Sons Ltd.

Is your anger justifiable because others agree with your reasons for being angry? Are you 'hanging on to your story' of why you're justified in being angry, as if your story can shield you from the need to let it go and move on?

Even though your anger is understandable because someone has behaved like a jerk, you can still choose to not be distressed with seething emotions. This is called insight. It can only be achieved by letting go of judgements. This letting go is not saying the person did the right thing. It's not even forgiveness, because some things people do to us are unforgiveable.

In order to remain angry at someone, you have to keep justifying it to yourself even subconsciously. The story of how they wronged you has to be told and retold again and again. It hurts every time, often subliminally.

So, you can see clearly that someone is a jerk and has not an iota of compassion in their body. But, by being insightful rather than judgemental, you are able to decide to not feel full of anger any more. This in turn allows you to not have to revisit the jerk's actions, seek revenge or allocate punishment. Their snide comments fly past you and have no effect on you because you have chosen to not be angry when you hear them. Choosing to be wise and non-reactionary frees you from the need to repeatedly tell your story. It can liberate you from an endless cycle of 'living the story' and telling the story so that others can reaffirm in you your perpetual anger and hatred.

> It's empowering to let go of anger, no matter how justified that anger is.

Have you noticed how, when you first met your partner/spouse/BFF, you thought good and positive thoughts about them, not only when you were spending time together, talking on the phone or texting them, but also when not present with them? You would have been thinking about their endearing personality, about the kind things they had done for you, listening to music you both like, planning fun nights out, etc.

All those thoughts *directly* contributed to your bond with that person and helped to build the relationship into something uplifting and positive.

Similarly, if the emotion you have chosen to observe is affection for someone close to you, build on it. Take that emotion and think about it further. Choose your internal and external reactions to it. Embrace the feelings of affection and kindness. Allow yourself to smile. The love grows as you feed it with your affectionate headspace.

Conversely, when we allow ourselves to seethe in anger, having negative thoughts about someone who has hurt us, when we spend hours having conversations in our heads with them, saying all the things we wished we'd said earlier, we create a monster of a character. And that monster makes us feel uncomfortable. The monster grows as we feed it with our angry headspace.

We all do it. And what a waste of time it is reliving the distressing past or, even worse, recreating a past conversation which never happened, isn't happening now and probably won't happen in the future.

That time could be spent so much more fruitfully.

Maybe the plan could be to simply not have conversations in your head. That conversation didn't happen, it isn't happening now and it is unlikely to happen in the future. Be mindful of the present and of the reality of the situation.

It's your choice if you want to do this or not. There's no rush.

The point here is that you are observing an emotion, naming it, looking it in the eye and then choosing your reaction. Even if you choose to stay angry for now. It's valid because it's your conscious decision.

Anxiety

Anxiety can be overwhelming. It can be crippling. It can destroy relationships and make us fail at work. It's often hard to pinpoint a single reason for our anxiety. It becomes our world. It's important to take the first steps of recognising it and naming it before then moving on to looking for its origin.

The physical symptoms of a racing heart and tight chest can cause further anxiety.

If you're feeling anxious, is it about something that has happened in the past or about something which may happen in the future? Are you able to pinpoint the source or sources of the anxiety?

For now, we are merely identifying (and not overidentifying with) the emotions.

Formulating a plan to deal with your anxiety can be so variable. It has to be tailored to your needs and to the individual causes.

Some people find that during a meditation, even identifying that anxiety is a powerful emotion within them causes more anxiety and their heart rate increases. The physical action of massaging the vagus nerve in your neck to lower your heart rate can help to regain focus. However, noticing the physical symptoms is a wonderful exercise in observing some of the effects that anxiety has on us.

Later in the book we will discuss how to sit with these feelings – physical and emotional.

Anxiety about a future event can be overpowering. We may find ourselves worrying about 10 potential outcomes of an event. Doing the maths, in reality, only one of those outcomes is going to happen. We will have wasted an enormous amount of time and mental energy worrying about the other nine. And we will be weaker as a result.

Planning for the future is essential if we are to be sensible citizens in the workplace, good parents, decent friends, of course. But worrying and stressing about it can occupy the part of our minds better used for increasing our mental strength in order that we can trust ourselves to be able to deal with whatever life throws at us, *when* it's thrown at us.

Learning to plan, without anxiety, for the short term and for the long term is a life skill worth cultivating.

For now, we are recognising and observing the emotion, naming it as anxiety and allowing it to pass until we're ready to tackle it.

> Learning to NOT ruminate and to NOT get drawn down into a spiral of increasing anxiety is probably one of the most helpful skills you can develop during these early stages of learning to meditate.

How to Meditate: Part 3

- Mini-meditations in the busy practice

Can you spare a minute? Can you spare five minutes?

If I said you could change your life if you could spare five minutes every day, would you do it?

Five-minute mini-meditations are for people who feel they are just are too busy for anything more. We have ridiculously busy lives. As vets and nurses, we multitask in our sleep.

Maybe we go to yoga once a week which is a formal way to practise mindfulness and that's great. However, what about the other days?

Everyone's talking about mindfulness for a reason. The benefits are immediate and multiple. It costs nothing. You can do it anywhere, in any clothes, at any time. So we can indeed meditate at work.

Mini-meditations are a calming, anxiety-relieving strategy which we can do at any time of the day.

> In every moment at work, there are infinite reasons to suffer and infinite reasons to be happy. What matters is where we're putting our attention.

While mini-meditations are a good place to start, they are essentially 'fire brigade treatment' for those of us experiencing a difficult time in our lives; a 'Band-Aid' until we make the time to use mindfulness more deeply.

There are literally thousands of meditation apps out there but proceed with caution. I would suggest instead disappearing somewhere quiet for five minutes *without* your phone, sit and focus on nothing other than your breathing. Toilet cubicles are an obvious place in a busy veterinary hospital. Closing your eyes while on the tube is another. Walking to work while concentrating on only your feet is another. It's much harder than you would think to maintain this clarity of concentration for a full five minutes.

Focus entirely on the present moment, your breathing, clear your mind of all thoughts which are trying to get your attention. Gently push

Mental Wellbeing and Positive Psychology for Veterinary Professionals: A Pre-emptive, Proactive and Solution-based Approach, First Edition. Laura Woodward.
© 2024 John Wiley & Sons Ltd. Published 2024 by John Wiley & Sons Ltd.

them to one side. Push the past to the left and the future to your right and concentrate fully on the here and now.

> To feel regretful, you need to be in the past; to worry you need to be in the future. But when you are fully in the present, you are momentarily free of regret and worry. That's like releasing a heavy burden for the duration of one breath or three breaths, allowing yourself half a minute of utter relief.

Once your mind is clear, then reintroduce and observe your emotions, in a direct and open manner, one at a time. Face each emotion, give it a description and a name. Be non-judgemental. No thought or emotion is right or wrong. Just accept it as the emotion it is. This is difficult. Once analysed, decide how much you want to hang onto or let go of that emotion. Then gently push that emotion aside. This is where you are powerful. Because you can literally choose the degree to which you feel that emotion from now on. If it is anger, you may wish to feel it less. If it is joy, you may wish to grow it so that it fills your mind for the day and makes you the person your colleagues want to work with.

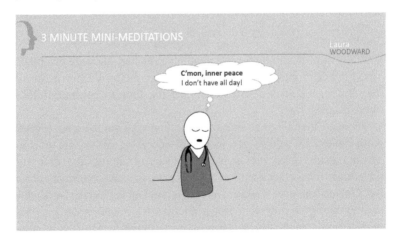

How to Meditate: Part 4

- Opening shutters meditation
- The fortress
- The heavy bucket
- Climbing up the branches of a tree
- Conveyor belt meditation

> By defusing troublesome thoughts, we can realise that they do not hold as much meaning and power over us as we thought they did.

So, by now, hopefully you are spending half an hour or more each morning being mindful and trying to achieve clarity. Then, observing emotions one at a time, giving them a name and thus defusing them to a degree. Formulating a plan to defuse the troublesome thoughts is a very personal thing, and as counsellors, we know that the best plans are those which you yourself devise. Contrary to popular belief, counsellors rarely advise a patient on what to do. Rather, we facilitate you in formulating your own plans and making your own decisions. Only then will the plan truly resonate with you, give you strength and teach you to tackle the many hurdles in your life without us, thus gaining more inner strength and improved self-esteem.

Similarly, the methods you choose to help you to gain clarity during meditation, to defuse those disturbing emotions and to become more compassionate are also very personal.

Here, I would like to share a few imagery methods which I and my patients have developed in order to help them with their practice.

Opening Shutters Meditation

It can be so hard to clear the mind so that we can even start. Some days will be easy and other days it will be impossible and that's okay. Every day is different, nothing stays the same and that is the nature of impermanence.

This is a nice imagery exercise to help you to clear your 'mind's eye'.

Mental Wellbeing and Positive Psychology for Veterinary Professionals: A Pre-emptive, Proactive and Solution-based Approach, First Edition. Laura Woodward.
© 2024 John Wiley & Sons Ltd. Published 2024 by John Wiley & Sons Ltd.

Get comfortable, sitting upright, eyes open or closed – it's up to you. Having a supportive cushion behind your back or your feet up of course is okay. This is your practice.

Imagine you are standing in front of a large window with the view hidden because there are heavy shutters closed and obscuring the view.

There's a chink of light between these shutters and you know the view beyond them is what you want to see.

It can be any view you pick. I nearly always want a view of the expansive calm ocean. Others want snow-covered mountains or the flat, white plains of Iceland. Maybe you even want to see your kids on the other side. In any case, all you can see at the moment is this chink of light.

Try to observe your breathing at the same time. This way, you have plenty to occupy your mind, so that it's a bit easier to not wander off into the past or the future.

Do whatever you like with this. Simply put, you are using your mind to help your mind.

Now imagine that the tall, heavy shutter on the left is all the stuff from the past. The distant past as well as what happened five minutes ago.

Pull as hard as you can to open that left shutter back a bit to clear your view of the beautiful outdoors.

Breathe in the view. Focus on it with all you've got.

Take a breath.

Now try to pull back the tall, heavy shutter on the right-hand side. This represents all the stuff in the future, things that need your attention. Not necessarily problems, just all the stuff you need to pay attention to after this meditation, later on today and next month.

Pull with all your might and make this view as large as you can.

Imagine you are holding both heavy shutters open with strength and focus on the clear view of what you've chosen.

See if you can focus on breathing in this view and little else.

Keep the shutters open for as long as you possibly can.

When the time comes, slowly close them one by one and remember that you can come back to this place whenever you want to have a clear mind.

The Fortress

Sometimes, people hurt us so much that we come to a decision to not engage with them again on an emotional level. One patient of mine came to this decision regarding her siblings who had spent as long as she could remember attacking her verbally and behind her back. Another member of her extended family had sexually abused her and her sister as children. She wanted to disempower them regarding their ability to hurt her any more. She wanted to be free of the hatred she felt towards them and to be liberated from them being in her thoughts constantly.

She built a fortress in her mind during meditation. The walls were so thick that no snide comment could get through. She could sense that her extended family were bad mouthing her, but she couldn't hear anything when within this fortress. The fortress had no roof though. Sunshine could come in and the skies above were blue and bright.

This was a short-term solution, of course. We cannot live life as an island, but when we gain strength, we can face our problems and unkind people without the fear of them hurting us. No, this was for her to get some space away from her spiteful siblings.

So, within the fortress, she gained strength through mindfulness. Soon, she could rise up to the top of the walls and look down on her family members who had hurt her so much for a lifetime. By this stage, she was so powerful emotionally that she could even wish them to be well, happy and peaceful. But they would never enter her mind during her meditations again which meant that they rarely entered her head during the weeks that followed.

The Heavy Bucket

Take that troublesome nagging thought, that disastrous day you had at work, that wound complication, that exam you failed, that parking fine and put all of them into a heavy bucket.

Raise your left arm out to your side to shoulder level, holding the bucket with the disastrous day in it. Feel it getting heavy, painful, festering. When you have decided that that entire day is in the bucket and you can feel the discomfort of the weight of it, drop it into the abyss, letting go. Put your hand back on your lap and concentrate on the physical and emotional relief of letting go of that stinking, heavy weight. It is the past. It doesn't need to be revisited or pondered upon any more. Stay with the feeling of extra space you have in your mind now that it has been dropped and let go. Feel the relief in your shoulder. Repeat with whatever imagery you wish.

Climbing Up the Branches of a Tree

Imagine you are feeling so many overwhelming emotions, you don't know where to start.

As we learnt earlier, clearing your mind to the point of being a blank canvas can be done. Observe one emotion at a time. Triage them.

We can imagine ourselves slowly ascending a tree to the top, which is our nirvana if you like. Each task on the way can be visualised as a branch on which you can rest and sunbathe and have a beer once you have tackled that challenge.

So, for example, I'm really angry with person X and that makes the first branch the place where I can rest once I have let go of the anger. We discussed methods of defusing anger in a previous chapter.

And here I am enjoying being free of the anger which was sapping my strength, resting on a branch enjoying my time.

The next branch above is even nicer, with more sunshine, a comfier sunbed and the beer is colder. But I have to conquer my fear and anxiety associated with person X in order to rise up to that branch.

It may take a week of meditation to get up onto the next branch. But each time you revisit your mindful meditation, you can start on the branch from where you let off the previous time.

Other branches up the tree can be named 'unbreakable', 'unshakeable', 'kind and compassionate to all' and finally 'true liberation and happiness'. Make it your own and it will have more meaning for you.

Conveyor Belt Meditation

This is a great one for when you're feeling overwhelmed with too much stuff in your head, numerous things to remember, a need for the mother of all multitasking to get through just the morning.

It feels counterintuitive to sit down and take 10 minutes when you don't have a minute to spare.

We all know the feeling at work of being about to tackle an urgent task only for someone to ask you to do something else at the same time. Then you sort that out but the first task is still needing to be done. The phone is hopping so you quickly answer it. Only it's never a quick call, is it? So, while you're organising whatever needs organising because of that call, you're still desperately trying to get the original task done and then there's an emergency, and an IT malfunction. The dryer is leaking and we've run out of drapes.

This is all made harder by the fact that everyone is being so nice in their requests and questions.

And it's not only at work. At home, there are mouths to feed: pets, people, you. The post needs to be dealt with, or at least opened, I still haven't sorted out my MOT which won't be any simpler than the phone calls at work. The laundry is now being renamed 'Mount Washmore' and apparently I'm supposed to be exercising and meditating for my wellbeing too.

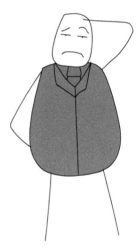

As always, sit comfortably and alertly, eyes open or closed.

Imagine all the 'stuff' you need to deal with and organise in a great big pile on the left. A plethora of lists all tangled up together.

Now imagine you're sitting in front of a conveyor belt onto which these items will be placed one by one.

Item one is placed on the belt, it moves into your line of view for a very short time and pauses. Just long enough for you to recognise what it is, e.g. book MOT.

This is non-judgemental. We're not looking to solve problems or do any actual sorting. Bear with me.

Next item comes into view. Look at it. Pause. Then it moves along and so on and on, with each individual item from this massive pile until there's nothing left.

When the pile is finished, keep an eye on the conveyor belt and notice its emptiness: it has run out of items.

Breathe for a while and appreciate the view of the empty place where the pile of things was.

When you are ready, open your eyes.

What many people say after this exercise is that they are surprised that the pile finishes at all. The list of things is actually finite. When it's a plethora of things, it feels unsurmountable. At least this way, we know it has an end.

This meditation can be the calming exercise that helps us to organise our time a bit more efficiently so that we actually, in reality, do get through some of the pile without becoming overwhelmed.

There will always be piles of things to do, and lists of tasks we need to tick off. We're lucky that we have a purpose, or many purposes, in life.

Feeling overwhelmed is normal and human, especially in the veterinary industry.

It doesn't have to be judged.

Part 3

Difficulties and Applying Strategies

> *It's your reaction to adversity as much as adversity itself that determines how your life story will develop.*
>
> Dieter F. Uchdorf

Anxiety

- Avoidance of anxiety
- Can anxiety be helpful?
- How to accept and live with anxiety

> *You can't stop the waves. But you CAN learn how to surf.*
>
> Jon Kabat-Zinn

The vast majority of my clients have said they are having trouble coming to terms with the levels of anxiety they are feeling.

Maybe they have always had a certain amount of unexplored anxiety running in the background and now it's come to the fore. Maybe they have a story which is causing them anxiety.

The fact is that feeling anxious is part of the human experience. Whether we have conquered problems in the past which were causing us concern, only for them to rear their ugly heads again many years later, or only recently discovered this phenomenon called anxiety which is novel to us, it's true to say that feeling anxiety is generally unpleasant.

So we avoid it. As a single-celled organism avoids a noxious substance, we avoid unpleasant thoughts, feelings and bodily sensations reflexively.

Most people describe a range of symptoms such as nausea, tight chest, tension in the jaw and shoulders, raised heart rate or palpitations and a lump in their throat.

Similarly, being self-aware and thus knowing what is likely to cause us fear and anxiety, we often avoid situations which will make us feel this way. Sensible, right?

Or, are we limiting ourselves and our experiences in life by avoiding these places, people and activities?

Wouldn't it be amazing if someone could wave a magic wand and make all those unpleasant feelings disappear, opening up a world of previously avoided opportunities for us?

Mental Wellbeing and Positive Psychology for Veterinary Professionals: A Pre-emptive, Proactive and Solution-based Approach, First Edition. Laura Woodward.
© 2024 John Wiley & Sons Ltd. Published 2024 by John Wiley & Sons Ltd.

Maybe life is just fine like this and the avoidance of potentially anxiety-ridden scenarios is working for you. There is no right or wrong degree of risk when it comes to placing yourself in the middle of uncomfortable emotions.

However, some of us may feel anxiety related to past situations which is recurrent, whether we like it or not. For example, ongoing health concerns which are unavoidable, people in our lives who are toxic and unavoidable, suboptimal employment issues. Maybe it's just the profession we're in.

And others would simply rather not feel limited by our fears and would like to be braver and more adventurous.

But is it the situation we fear? Or are we afraid of feeling anxious? If it's the latter, why are we afraid of an emotion?

Mindfulness practice is about being totally present in the current moment, on purpose. But what if the current moment is a godawful crisis? What if the current moment is causing me anxiety and I don't know why?

Being present with our emotions and thoughts is not just about truly appreciating the wonderful moments in life before they pass by. It's about noticing the thoughts however pleasant or awful they are, and being aware of their influence on us, our minds and our bodies.

So, during your mindfulness practice, allowing yourself to feel anxious can be surprisingly therapeutic. We already know that the act of feeling an emotion, looking it in the face and giving it a name defuses its hold on us. It is possible to take that a bit further in our mindfulness practice.

Jon Kabat-Zinn describes this venture into uncomfortable feelings as dipping our toe into cold water. You know how it is – you dip a toe in, you become acclimatised to the unpleasant feelings and then you put your foot in. Soon, both feet are in and then you very slowly wade in up to your knees or even take the plunge and swim. 'It's okay once you're in.'

Similarly, when sitting on the cushion or wherever else you choose to meditate, really getting dug into this emotion and these feelings of sickness in your stomach can be a 'dipping in of your toe' and acclimatising yourself to these uncomfortable sensations, further liberating you from their grip. Because their grip on us is greater when we try to put them in a box compared to when we stand face to face looking at them.

For those feeling very brave, while meditating, try to become aware of your racing pulse, your hyperpnoea; really be at one with that feeling that you want to throw up. Hold that thought and dive in.

And then, maybe, just maybe, it's not so bad once you're in.

A rapid heart rate and a lurching of your stomach are unpleasant, for sure. But are they to be feared to such a degree that you limit your life choices to avoid them at all costs?

With each scenario which you know will cause you anxiety, it's worth asking yourself 'Is it the scenario I'm afraid of? Or is it the emotions I fear?'

It is for each of us to decide how much (if at all) we want to change the hold that anxiety has on us. There is no right or wrong in this practice.

You might be tempted to avoid the messiness of daily living for the tranquility of stillness and peacefulness. This of course would be an attachment to stillness, and like any strong attachment, it leads to delusion. It arrests development and short-circuits the cultivation of wisdom.

Jon Kabat-Zinn

Fear of Failure

- The Dalai Lama advises
- How do I stop fearing fear?
- Disputing irrational beliefs and doing our cognitive homework
- Change your language in order to change your thought process
- Exercises for attacking shame
- Imagery and role play
- Desensitisation
- Skills training

Fear of failure is common in new and recent graduates, many of whom have never failed at anything in their lives before. These people have been getting A*s since primary school and now they enter the workplace where small failures are part of everyday work and life.

The terror associated with failure can be overwhelming at a pivotal time in their career, and many vets and nurses leave their professions at this stage because of the insomnia and stress associated with this difficulty.

> "But there's no release, no peace. I toss and turn without cease. Like a curse, open my eyes, rise like yeast. At least a couple of weeks since I last slept" Faithless - Insomnia.

When the word 'fail' changes from being a verb, 'I might fail at that', to becoming a noun, 'I am a failure', then we are verging on *atychiphobia* or a phobia of failure.

As vets and nurses, a healthy fear of failure makes us strive for the best clinical outcome. However, when we are so gripped with this fear that we lose sleep, avoid bitch spays, leave the CRI calculations to someone more experienced or procrastinate about interventional treatments, then we are doing our patients and ourselves a disservice.

When researching the plethora of self-help guides for non-veterinary professionals on how to overcome fear of failure, so many advise us to 'Give it a go', 'Believe in yourself', 'Only through failure can we gain knowledge'.

Mental Wellbeing and Positive Psychology for Veterinary Professionals: A Pre-emptive, Proactive and Solution-based Approach, First Edition. Laura Woodward.
© 2024 John Wiley & Sons Ltd. Published 2024 by John Wiley & Sons Ltd.

The Dalai Lama Advises

Fear is the mind killer, the eradicator of potential and the eraser of personal progress.

Dalai Lama

If you are afraid because you have no self-confidence and feel that nothing you do will ever succeed, stop a while to think it over. Try to see why you imagine you are a loser before you have even started. The problem stems from your way of thinking, not from real ineptitude.

Given that the Dalai Lama isn't referring to vets or vet nurses here, where failure can actually be catastrophic, it can be hard to apply this insight to our situation. 'Giving it a go' is unacceptable and immoral when you're in our professions.

Having said that, often the problem does indeed stem from our way of thinking more than from past failures. By changing the way we think, we can change the way we feel and therefore change our actions.

How Do I Stop Fearing Fear?

And then, how do I stop fearing failure? All the while knowing that I have a moral obligation to work within my abilities and can never just 'give it a go'.

Where do we draw the line?

I use Acceptance and Commitment Therapy (ACT; see Part Four, Chapter 3) with mindfulness to help to rationalise our fear of failure, whilst keeping us practising responsibly and ethically.

Instead of repressing or avoiding the procedures or interventions which we fear, in ACT the focus is placed on accepting the feeling of being fearful but still taking action, i.e. tackling the fear head on.

Fear is a conception. A valid feeling but nevertheless it is an emotion.

Other times I use Cognitive Behavioural Therapy (CBT; see Part Four, Chapter 1) to relieve the anxiety associated with fear of failure in a particular situation.

For example, if spaying an overweight Labrador is a procedure you would never tackle for fear of failing, and supposing that fear is paralysing you, let's make a list of all the things that could go wrong during this procedure. It's a long list.

Now rate each complication according to likelihood, being as objective as you can be.

Your stomach may be lurching now.

Next to each complication, you could write what actions you should take to rectify the situation. All the while, you are facing your fears head on and no patient is at risk.

Role play can help. With your eyes closed, you can 'walk' your way through the whole procedure, ligatures slipping, bleeders happening, blood pressure dropping, etc.

You can also walk yourself through rectifying these one by one with as much true imagination as you can. Try to imagine the anxiety you would feel at the same time and see if you can simulate the physical symptoms these complications give rise to within you.

Or, if you are a recently qualified nurse, and the fear of this anaesthetic going wrong is making you pass it to someone else rather than increasing your skill set, I advise you to use similar concepts.

Make a list of the anaesthetic complications and rate them in order of likelihood.

Make a plan for each complication and see if you can role play your way through each one along with the nausea and tight chest.

The most experienced anaesthetists usually have a list of pressors, blood products and other drugs written up prior to a procedure as a normal way of working, so this exercise isn't so misplaced.

Let's apply a few basic CBT concepts to our situation.

Disputing Irrational Beliefs and Doing Our Cognitive Homework

Instead of believing that if we spay that bitch, she will bleed out and die, try to be rational about the chances of that patient actually bleeding out and dying. Yes, there is that risk. However, it may be minimal. Even in your hands.

Try to think rationally about the following points.

- How many spays have you performed?
- How many times have you had bleeding vessels with spays?
- How many times have you found a bleeding vessel and ligated it?
- How much supervision do you have?
- How safe is this patient if you become frozen or unable to rectify an emergency?

I can't answer these questions for you and the answers will be different for everyone. It's about stopping, pausing and trying to see mathematically if your beliefs match up with the facts.

As the nurse, what could potentially go wrong? Would you recognise a problem? How many different monitoring techniques are you experienced with?

What could you do in each scenario?

Do you have supervision and a capable person to consult if you become unable to do this safely?

For vet and nurse, maybe this patient is, in fact, in real danger in your hands. Maybe this patient is in no danger because you will do a safe procedure or because you have an experienced person available to alleviate danger at all times.

> Is your fear rational? Or exaggerated? Figuring out the answer to this question is what can keep this patient safe and help you to think clearly and methodically while advancing your skills.

Change Your Language in Order to Change Your Thought Process

Instead of 'I'm not spaying that bitch because she will bleed to death', try saying 'I will spay that bitch. However, I may need help if she starts to bleed'. In this way, we are changing from a 'can't do' attitude to a 'can do with supervision' attitude and putting a strategy in place in case our fears are realised.

Use clear communication. For example, instead of 'I've never done an anaesthetic like that', you could say 'This is a challenge for me. I need someone to monitor me'.

Maybe it is semantics but using positive language in our heads or out loud can have a profound effect on our ability to upskill.

If we upskill at no risk to our patients, then that is a positive move.

Exercises for Attacking Shame

There is little to be gained from feeling shameful because we aren't 'up to the job'. Try to steer away from self-flagellation.

It's easy to believe that we are rubbish at anaesthesia and surgery if we say it to ourselves in our heads. In fact, it's easier to believe the negative views we have than any positive self-affirmations.

If, however, you feel you are a danger to a patient, then it is acting in a professional and ethical manner to say it. We cannot 'have a go' in the hope we get better whatever the risks.

So, if after doing our cognitive homework and identifying that, in fact, our fears are rational, i.e. 'I am not capable of keeping that patient safe' for whatever reasons, we pass that case to someone more experienced, it is essential to stop ourselves from spiralling into a negative follow-on exercise.

By this, I mean that 'I'm not capable of keeping this patient safe this time' can be the end of it. Or it can be the beginning of learning how to keep patients like this safe in the future.

That is a positive for everyone.

Spiralling into 'I'm useless', 'I'll never be any good at this', 'I'm a burden and bothering my colleagues' is what we call self-shaming. We often do this. Sometimes, it may be because we're seeking affirmation from our colleagues who send reassuring responses our way. But it's not a healthy habit to speak to yourself that way. What does it achieve?

You wouldn't speak to your colleague like that, so why are you saying it to yourself?

Learning to stop this spiral is an essential life skill. Being aware of where the spiral starts is difficult.

Imagery and Role Play

I, and many other surgeons, will play out a procedure in our minds before the actual event. It helps to plan and to focus. It might be useful, prior to the bitch spay, to imagine the procedure from incision to closure. Then imagine it including the ligature slip and bleeding and visualise yourself finding the vessel and ligating it.

Similarly, imagining and acting out your actions if the anaesthetic goes in different directions is pre-emptive, wise and calming.

Desensitisation

It may be stating the obvious, but the more often you spay large bitches (albeit with someone more experienced available to scrub in if necessary), the less it will frighten you. Of course, the more often you tackle a bleeding pedicle, the easier it will become also. If you can, whenever you are successfully doing a procedure, it's a helpful exercise to be aware that something could have gone wrong. Ask yourself what you would do. Feel the rush of adrenaline and the anxiety, the stomach lurching and the heart sinking feeling.

Desensitisation means exposing yourself to a stimulus so it causes less of a reaction in the future. So, becoming accustomed to heightened awareness and the adrenaline rush of theatre means that you are less like to freeze when a real emergency arises in the future.

Skills Training

There are many CPD providers running wet labs for surgery. Try to get immersed in these emotionally as well as physically. Treat them like they are real cases and feel the sensations that come with that while seeing that you can still operate effectively while stressed.

CPD for veterinary nurses has evolved over the years to be something fantastic.

Online webinars, in-person lectures and wet labs for nurses are all readily available now.

When a difficult anaesthetic comes in, maybe you can shadow the anaesthetist, then be shadowed, then do it by yourself, albeit with someone ready outside the theatre door.

Actioning these progressions can be daunting, especially in a busy practice. Be courageous and try to make it happen.

To overcome the fear of failure, do what makes you fearful.

Debasish Mridha

Loss of Confidence

A loss of faith in one's ability happens frequently, especially after a significant or catastrophic failure. Sometimes it takes years to become 'unstuck' and many choose to pull back from responsibilities such as surgery or anaesthesia at this stage.

Loss of confidence can affect any one of us at every stage of our careers. It's not a new graduate 'thing'. It's not a specialist 'thing'. It can occur for any reason or no reason. But being unaware of this or being unprepared is avoidable if we practise good mental wellbeing exercises.

Loss of confidence in one's abilities can happen to the best of the best. Sometimes, when we're at the top of our game, we feel that we've reached the pinnacle and that it will be this way forever. Thinking that we can never lose that position at the top of our game is to be in denial that it can happen to us as well. Sometimes with disastrous consequences and even suicide.

I spoke to a prominent veterinary orthopaedic specialist at a conference last year. He was someone whom I had always admired for his practical surgical solutions, and especially after a weekend where we had talked about nothing but surgical complications all holed-up in a relatively small room in a hotel. It was an intense course.

It made us realise that complications happen, and we had to be prepared for them and ready to apply a belt-and-braces approach to revising and repairing them.

This man clearly accepted a lot about not just orthopaedics but life as well. He was in his late 40s when he noticed his eyesight was starting to change, as happens to many people. He tried various ways of improving his vision but to no avail. He decided to change his path from specialist at the top of his game to freelance management.

He wasn't regretful, he was happy, content with his life path, present and mindful. He wasn't rehashing the past or worrying about the future, he was enjoying the conference and our conversation. This was a man applying his belt-and-braces approach to the lack of permanence which is inevitable in life, eyesight, the veterinary world. I admired him even more after that day.

Mental Wellbeing and Positive Psychology for Veterinary Professionals: A Pre-emptive, Proactive and Solution-based Approach, First Edition. Laura Woodward.
© 2024 John Wiley & Sons Ltd. Published 2024 by John Wiley & Sons Ltd.

If we are resistant to ageing, eyesight changes or arthritis in our fingers, our pain when they happen will be greater, not less.

Several surgeons in the UK, veterinary and human, have been so resistant to change happening, so in denial about the physical changes in their hands, that the decrease in their surgical ability has caused such loss of confidence and terror that they have taken their own lives.

Suicide has multiple precursors and no two suicide victims are the same. Loss of confidence and decreasing expertise are two possible precursors.

Realising that loss of confidence can affect any one of us, even if we are currently the best of the best, is wisdom.

Perfectionism

Still identifying with the life of high achievement we've had prior to entering the workplace, perfectionism can be paralysing to us, unhelpful to our colleagues, and unrealistic and misleading to the clients.

Becoming non-judgemental liberates us from the habit of hiding our mistakes and retreating behind self-deprecation. It allows us to acknowledge our errors, to face them and all the emotions they give rise to, and to feel shame, embarrassment and agony in all their fullness so that we can move on.

This is learning how to *not* be a perfectionist. We don't learn this at school or at college. It's alien to most of us.

Striving to be the best vet, nurse, person you can be is always an asset to the practice, your friends and loved ones, right? Not necessarily so.

When striving to be great is accompanied by a yearning to be better than we realistically can be, it's a perfect storm that can lead us into a destructive circle of yearning, being disappointed, self-judgement, self-flagellation, trying harder, more disappointment, more harsh judgement, loneliness and desperation.

Now, I'm not saying we should stop trying to be the best we can be. Not at all. But so many of my therapy clients who are self-declared recovering perfectionists find that swapping the above cycle for a less judgemental one means that they have the head space to focus more clearly on tasks at work, thus leading to better outcomes for their patients, colleagues and ultimately their clients and their pets. Ironically, accepting less than perfection can improve their quality of work.

Have you ever been with someone who constantly puts themselves down, listing their own faults, errors and inabilities in an effort to convince their audience that they are worthless?

Or have you ever been that person?

Mental Wellbeing and Positive Psychology for Veterinary Professionals: A Pre-emptive, Proactive and Solution-based Approach, First Edition. Laura Woodward.
© 2024 John Wiley & Sons Ltd. Published 2024 by John Wiley & Sons Ltd.

And have you ever been in the company of someone who accepts that they aren't infallible, who owns their imperfections and makes sure those imperfections don't impact on their patients, colleagues or friends?

Who would you rather be with? Who would you rather be?

For me, I feel more confident in my colleague's ability to handle a case if they realise their limitations and ask for help rather than forging ahead when the risk of errors is high.

And when something goes wrong with a case, again a colleague who takes ownership of the complication, focuses on the patient and deals with it, with or without help from others, is much more valuable than someone who self-flagellates out loud, listing their incompetencies and being eloquent about how rubbish they are, i.e. focusing away from the patient and onto themselves.

So, how can we not beat ourselves up when faced with a complication at work, or when faced with what we see as a flaw in our general make-up?

Being ambitious and always wanting to do better while not trying to be perfect are qualities we want in our vets and nurses. As surgeons, we are encouraged to criticise our work and learn reflectively every time we operate. What five things could I have done better on this fracture repair? Even if we are happy with our repair and we know that the outcome is likely to be a comfortable leg and a rapid return to normal function, developing a healthy habit of self-assessment does so much for us as surgeons and as people outside work.

So, what's the difference between self-assessment and being judgemental when faced with a complication or when we have failed to some degree? It may seem subtle, nuanced or even non-existent until examined more closely.

Jon Kabat-Zinn defines mindfulness as 'the awareness that arises from paying attention, on purpose, in the present moment and non-judgmentally'.

Non-judgementally broadly means not putting any thought or emotion into a 'good' category or a 'bad' category but rather just noticing it, accepting it and allowing ourselves to feel it.

Non-judgement isn't always about judging people or things they have done or their characteristics. Nor is it about judging ourselves. It's about relieving ourselves of the need to place things into boxes. So, situations, thoughts, emotions, people, even the weather can just be.

An easy starter for this is a simple mini-meditation on non-judgement.

So, sitting comfortably, eyes open or shut, take 10 normal breaths, noticing only the movement of the breath in and out of the nose.

If a thought comes into your head during this time, gently push it aside for now.

Then, during your body scan which we have practised in previous chapters, try to notice any discomforts. For example, you may have an itchy scalp or an aching joint. You might be sitting not quite comfortably enough. Maybe you would rather change your posture.

Then, without scratching the itch or moving the uncomfortable position, try to notice the physical feelings associated with it.

Name the physical sensations. It might be 'itchy', 'irritated', 'painful', etc.

Allow them to be, without doing anything to relieve the discomfort or annoyance. Focus on the discomfort wholeheartedly. It doesn't need to be perfect.

That is acceptance of discomfort and acceptance of imperfection.

You can open your eyes and try to notice the relief of not having to correct the imperfections.

A mini-meditation for when we have failed is harder.

Again, close your eyes and clear your mind to make space for this meditation (e.g. breath meditation, body scan meditation).

Instead of feeling just the physical discomforts, we feel the emotional pain of failing. Many emotions come to mind: shame, embarrassment, self-doubt, loneliness, desperation.

We may tend towards *awfulisation*, where the potential outcomes of our error become enormous in our mind and tend towards the worst possible scenario as a definite reality.

Physically, we might feel nauseous, weak or faint. Or we might have palpitations, a sinking feeling in our chest or a lurching stomach. We've all been there.

The challenge of this meditation is to allow these feelings to be present one by one in the forefront of your mind for as long as you can hold them there. It's difficult when our natural reaction is to push these hideous feeling away.

Once you've seen an emotion associated with the failure, named it and felt it for as long as you can, allow it to pass to make room for the next emotion. Keep doing this until you feel you've reached the end of the queue.

Return to a breath meditation for a few minutes before you open your eyes.

It has been shown time and time again that naming feelings, whether it's the feeling of nausea or the emotion of shame, looking them in the eye and allowing yourself to feel them at their fullest defuses their hold on you, thus enabling you to get on with your life.

It is so important to pull your mind away from trying to justify why you feel any of these feelings. Therein lies the non-judgement part. It doesn't matter if you should or shouldn't feel a feeling. The point is that you do feel it and that's it.

Now is not the time for yearning for the error to not have happened. It has happened. So, when we're being non-judgemental of the emotions we're feeling as a result of not being perfect, we are indeed noticing them, allowing ourselves to feel them and accepting that they exist.

We aren't justifying whether these feeling should or shouldn't exist. We aren't defending to anyone why we're feeling what we're feeling.

We're just noticing each emotion one by one, looking it in the eyes and giving it a name. Recognising that the plethora of feelings can indeed be sorted into an orderly queue of individual emotions, dealt with and accepted. Like the mass of cables behind the TV, when untangled, it's a great deal easier to organise them.

> Isn't it telling that when we make a mistake in our professions, it's called '*committing* an error'? Similar to committing a crime or committing a murder.

Dealing with errors in a team which runs morbidity and mortality rounds is a fantastic way to learn how to accept imperfections and mistakes. Like a mini-meditation but as a group of fallible beings.

Morbidity and mortality rounds, when run intelligently, are an opportunity to say out loud that something went wrong, and we did it. Then it's out in the open. These rounds aren't about blaming anyone, we all know who did what. It's about accepting that we make errors and that there are outcomes from these errors. We talk about the near misses and the deaths that we didn't prevent. We feel sick to the core when talking about it. The physical feelings and the emotion of shame are a given. We feel them as a team. We discuss how to prevent various mistakes from happening again, put more protocols in place and, ironically, we come away from these meetings even more bonded as a team and more at peace with the fact that we made those mistakes, they make us feel hideous and that's life in the veterinary world.

Imposter Syndrome

- Feel like a fraud?
- What can I do?
- Recognise your expertise
- Remember what you do well
- Talk about it

Feel Like a Fraud?

Many of my clients feel that they have achieved good results at work due to chance or good luck.

Imposter syndrome occurs when there is a mismatch between our abilities and our confidence. It is a lonely place to be, with irrationalities and internal chatter being unhelpful. Imposter syndrome occurs amongst high achievers who are unable to internalise and accept their success. They feel that they are a fraud and about to be 'found out' instead of being able to celebrate their well-earned successes, big and small. In essence, they strived, they achieved and they were left anxious and empty.

Many vets and vet nurses in counselling have said to me 'I'm a fraud, and everyone is about to find out'. Either they have been successful at work, or maybe they've made a small error which, when discovered, will reveal their other errors and uncover how incompetent they really are.

While fear of failure is rife amongst our newer graduates, feeling like a fraud or 'imposter syndrome' is more common amongst those of us who graduated a little longer (e.g. two to four years out) and are wondering why on earth the fractures we treat are healing, or how we are 'getting away with it' when our cardiac failure patients are feeling great or our geriatrics are eating.

First described by psychologist Suzanne Imes, PhD, in the 1970s, imposter syndrome occurs among high achievers who are unable to internalise and accept their success. By definition, most people suffering from imposter syndrome suffer in silence. Most don't talk about it. Part of the experience is that they're afraid they're going to be found out, Yet

Mental Wellbeing and Positive Psychology for Veterinary Professionals: A Pre-emptive, Proactive and Solution-based Approach, First Edition. Laura Woodward.
© 2024 John Wiley & Sons Ltd. Published 2024 by John Wiley & Sons Ltd.

I would estimate that 50% of my clients have experienced it at some stage of their careers, so it's not uncommon.

How does imposter syndrome get out of hand? The trigger is often perfectionism. In its mild form, a healthy degree of perfectionism provides the energy that can lead to great accomplishments clinically. Of course, this is desirable as we are, after all, looking after living beings and we don't want to learn from our mistakes.

'Benign perfectionists', who do not suffer feelings of imposter syndrome, derive pleasure from their achievements and don't obsess over failures. 'Neurotic imposters', however, cannot appreciate their achievements as anything but a stroke of luck.

Many people who feel like imposters grow up in families that place a big emphasis on achievement, in particular with parents who send mixed messages, alternating between overpraise and criticism. This can increase the risk of future fraudulent feelings.

> Alternating between overpraise and criticism can increase the risk of future fraudulent feelings.

There can be a lot of confusion between approval, love and worthiness. Self-worth becomes contingent on achieving, says Innes.

So, as parents, it is our duty to attach our children's self-worth to more than just accomplishments and successes. A well rounded contented person knows how to have fun, how to be unsuccessful, how to fail and learn from that experience with support from their colleagues and friends, how to enjoy learning even if there is no grade to achieve at the end.

What Can I Do?

With effort, you can stop feeling like a fraud and learn to enjoy your accomplishments.

Often, vets and nurses affected by imposter feelings don't realise they could be living some other way. They don't have any idea that it's possible to not feel so anxious and fearful all the time.

Recognise Your Expertise

Teaching younger students or new graduates is an instant way to boost your confidence and realise that you have indeed got knowledge and expertise.

Remember What You Do Well

Write a list of what you do well. Now write a list of what you don't (yet) do well. There, your secret's in the open. The burden of shame and secrecy is decreased.

Talk About It

Be the person in your practice who instigates monthly morbidity and mortality rounds, where mistakes in patient care are openly discussed without blame, in order to establish protocols to help avoid a recurrence. In his book Complications, Atul Gawande describes M and M rounds as a sombre process designed to discourage self doubt and also to decrease shame. Self doubt after a failure can lead to loss of confidence as we described previously. Shame is common after we do something incorrectly or fail to do what's correct. By putting our failures as individuals and as a group out there and speaking about them, our abilities can be measured by more experienced colleagues and it isn't a secret anymore. We get an objective view of where we are on the scale of abilities and we're no longer an imposter. Then we can truly enjoy our successes with the knowledge they didn't happen by chance.

In this way, not only are you facing your own imposter syndrome head on and thus negating its effect on you, you are helping all your other colleagues secretly suffering from the same syndrome to face their demons and rise above them. That's a real achievement, not one born out of pure luck.

Compassion Fatigue

- What are the symptoms of compassion fatigue?
- How do I prevent or recover from compassion fatigue?

One of the greatest strengths that we have to bring to our occupation – our capacity to develop a compassionate connection with our clients – is also our greatest vulnerability.

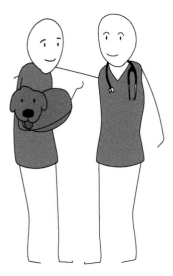

Depersonalisation and numbness are components of compassion fatigue. This is one of the recognisable stepping stones on the path to burnout.

Most of us became vets and nurses out of a love of animals and a desire to help them. But a love of humans was not listed as a prerequisite for our career choice. Sometimes we love them, sometimes we're stressed by them, sometimes we shut ourselves off from their emotions as an act of self-preservation.

Nevertheless, the more we 'love' the people who are tethered to our patients, the more job satisfaction we are likely to have. This is particularly true when fixing fractures, obstructions of any system, chronic co-morbidities of geriatric patients and long-term inpatients requiring intensive nursing care.

If we can celebrate with the owners of our patients, then it's all good, right? However, the downside to having a close emotional bond with our clients is that, without good self-awareness and self-regulation, we can feel their emotions a bit too intensely. We can 'become' their emotions of fear when investigations are being discussed, and grief and sadness when things aren't going well.

This in turn saps our strength, and leaves nothing in the tank for actually doing what the client wants us to do: diagnose and treat.

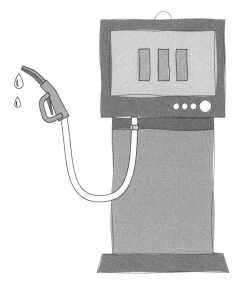

Our capacity for compassion, on top of the insanely busy days and other emotional strains can lead to emotional exhaustion and compassion fatigue.

So, is shutting off from others the solution? No. This only serves to increase our vulnerability. This is because being a rock and an island is only ever a temporary 'fix'. Humans need positive relationships in order to thrive.

There is an abundance of literature showing that people who are socially integrated and who experience more supportive and rewarding relationships with others have better mental health, higher levels of subjective wellbeing and lower rates of morbidity and mortality compared to others (Minkler 1985).

Even more interestingly, one meta-analysis (Holt-Lunstad and Smith 2012) shows that being socially integrated in a network of meaningful relationships predicts mortality *more* strongly than many lifestyle behaviours (e.g. smoking, physical activity), i.e. the better the relationships, the lower the mortality rate in middle age.

What are the Symptoms of Compassion Fatigue?

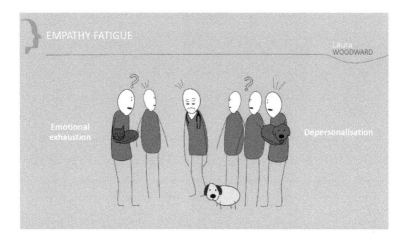

Compassion fatigue and PTSD have many symptoms in common.

- Depersonalisation (isolation from others, feeling like a zombie or an onlooker onto your own life).
- Difficulty falling asleep or staying asleep.
- Feeling like you're never refreshed when you wake up.
- Irritability.
- Hopeless attitude towards your job.
- Feeling like you have to just 'get through' each day.
- Difficulty in leaving work at the end of the day.
- Thinking about cases when not at work.
- Dreaming about cases.

- 'Awfulising' about cases (an irrational and dramatic thought pattern characterised by the tendency to overestimate the potential bad outcomes of a case). Predicting the most catastrophic outcome.

How Do I Prevent or Recover from Compassion Fatigue?

Awareness of the symptoms and *early recognition* are crucial. Using mindfulness to enhance self-awareness will alert us to the difference between having good empathy with a client and having 'too much' empathy with them.

Self-regulation: knowing when the drain on your emotional resources is more than what is being replenished *as it's happening* in the consult room or on the phone. And being able to stop yourself travelling down that emotional spiral with your distressed client in order to stay strong.

Relating to our pet owners with empathy and sincerity makes being a vet and nurse so much more rewarding than if we didn't care about them. However, it is possible to have *too* much empathy so that we are left running on empty emotionally because we have given too much without realising.

I like to use this wine bottle analogy when talking about too much empathy.

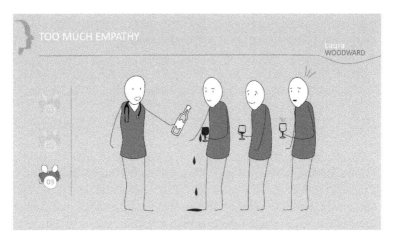

If I have a bottle of wine and I know that there is a queue of people who need a glass of this wine, if I overfill the first person's glass, there isn't much left for the next person's glass and the last person gets no wine at all. Not only that, what's left for me?

It's better to notice the level of wine in the bottle as you are pouring it slowly and check it in between each glass so that you don't end up with nothing for yourself.

Through self-awareness and self-regulation, you can stop, pause and take a look at how you are feeling right now. It only takes a moment. Then, you can decide how much you have left in the tank before you end up running on empty. Armed with this real-time knowledge, you can still be empathic, kind, caring and professional.

What you will be avoiding is oversharing, oversympathising and emotional exhaustion.

Taking time off doesn't necessarily bring relief for many of us, either because we're thinking about work and checking our emails while we're off, or because we return to the workplace having done little to no self-care whilst away.

A holiday can still be a holiday even if we're getting the 'chore' of self-compassion done.

Self-care and self-compassion ideally shouldn't be at the bottom of our 'to do' list, only to be ignored when we've finished work because we're exhausted, or avoided when on holiday because 'we need a break'.

Making time for short mindful meditations each and every day provides a structure for psychological self-care. Make that 10 minutes or half hour non-negotiable with your self-neglecting self.

> *My mission in life is not merely to survive, but to thrive; and to do so with some passion, some compassion, some humour, and some style. Surviving is important. Thriving is elegant.*
>
> Maya Angelou

We all know that *good nutrition, good sleep and exercise* are helpful. I don't know any vet or nurse who's nailed this. Maybe this could be adjusted for each of us to make it realistic and achievable, e.g. slightly less than a bottle of wine, no screens just before bedtime and walking some of the way to work. Whatever plan you make, stick to it. Because if it's your own plan, it's a great deal more valid than a plan your therapist has made for you.

Invest in your *positive relationships* and nurture them with more than just text messages and Facebook posts. Spend time with the people who feed your soul, refill your tank, and who genuinely care about you. Put your phone on silent somewhere else when you're with them if you can. Spend *less time with the negative influences* in your life.

Unrecognised and untreated compassion fatigue causes vets and nurses to leave the profession, hit the bottle or in all too many cases become self-destructive or suicidal. Recognising the symptoms in ourselves and our colleagues benefits everyone: those with emotional exhaustion, those trying to avoid it, the clients we see, and the animals we treat.

> *Taking care of myself doesn't mean 'me first', it means 'me too'.*
>
> L. R. Knost

References

Holt-Lunstad, J. and Smith, T.B. (2012). Social relationships and mortality. *Social and Personality Psychology Compass.* https://doi.org/10.1111/j.1751-9004.2011.00406.x.

Minkler, M. (1985). Social support and health of the elderly. In: *Social Support and Health* (ed. S. Cohen and S.L. Syme), 199–216. New York: Academic Press.

Lack of Assertiveness

- Empathy
- Motivation

> *Are we human? Or are we dancer?*
>
> Brandon Flowers, The Killers

> Assertiveness is a social skill which relies heavily on effective communication whilst always taking into account the thoughts and feelings of others.
>
> www.psychologytoday.com/us/basics/assertiveness

I don't disagree with this at all. I do have a concern, though, that 'always taking into account the thoughts and feelings of others' neglects the essential elements of self-care and self-compassion we need if we are to survive. Assertiveness needs communication skills, empathy and self compassion to all be running in sync if it is to be effective.

Often, we are promoted to a higher position simply through longevity at the practice or because we are effective communicators and excellent clinicians. Having most of the attributes of emotional intelligence (self-awareness, self-regulation, motivation, empathy and social skills) is frequently what gets us noticed, valued and promoted by management.

But if we lack that essential skill of motivation at full throttle, it's easy to see why being 'responsibly selfish' (as I've described before in the discussion on motivation) gets put on the back burner.

So, what does 'responsibly selfish' mean? If 'selfishness' is socially unacceptable, how can putting the word 'responsibly' in front of it make it okay? Furthermore, how can that help me or others in a position of management have a better life in and out of work?

Motivation, the third component of emotional intelligence, means 'what do I want out of this situation and how can I achieve that?'. It's okay to want something. We talked about judgement and self-judgement in earlier chapters.

Mental Wellbeing and Positive Psychology for Veterinary Professionals: A Pre-emptive, Proactive and Solution-based Approach, First Edition. Laura Woodward.
© 2024 John Wiley & Sons Ltd. Published 2024 by John Wiley & Sons Ltd.

The self-judgement that arises within us when we are being responsibly selfish reactively hammers that thought of self-care on the head and puts it back where we believe it belongs: in the box with the lid shut. Selfish is 'bad' and selfless is 'good', right?

Maybe we should pause, breathe and take a good look at these emotions before slamming that lid shut.

First, a quick recap on the five competencies of emotional intelligence.

Self-awareness (in a nutshell) means I am aware of how I am feeling now, how I've felt in the past, how I am likely to feel in a given situation, and I am aware of my strengths and limitations.

Self-regulation is my ability to pause and choose my reaction internally and externally to a given situation or emotion.

> *Between a stimulus and response there is a space. In that space is our power to choose our response. In our response lies our growth and our freedom.*
>
> Viktor Frankl

Motivation is deciding what I want out of a given situation and figuring out how I can achieve that. It's worth noting here that what I want out of a given situation might be joy and happiness for someone else.

Empathy is broadly divided into cognitive empathy, emotional empathy and empathic concern. Cognitive empathy means I understand what you are saying and what you are communicating without words, and I can communicate with you in a way which will relate to you. Emotional empathy means I understand what you are feeling, and I feel your distress and also your joy. I can see things from your perspective. Empathic concern means I feel your pain and I have an overwhelming need to help you out.

Social skills include eye contact, body language, active listening, etc.

So here's the thing . . . feeling some self-loathing because you're reacting to looking at yourself in the mirror while feeling 'selfish' is a worthwhile exercise.

Feel the negativity you are directing at yourself because you're trying to get something out of a situation.

Notice the self-flagellation resulting from wanting to survive and to enjoy your job.

Listen to you berating yourself for moaning.

Now, imagine your friend is the person who wants to enjoy their job. Picture them running on empty. Watch others fire clinical questions and holiday requests at them until they break. What would you say to that friend? Would it be 'Power on through', 'Turn that frown upside down', 'Always take into account the thoughts and feelings of others' or 'It's just because you're tired'? I'm guessing not. It's unlikely to be helpful and it's ignoring the fundamental problem which is lack of true self-compassion and lack of responsible selfishness.

Empathy

If we choose to really engage with cognitive empathy, we are probably already pretty good at communicating ideas to others. However, now you're asking for something for yourself, ask yourself this: 'Am I communicating my distress to those around me or just hoping they'll suss it out?'.

If we pride ourselves on emotional empathy, are we really walking a mile in someone else's shoes? Have we really made the effort to see where they are coming from with the barrage of emails, questions, texts and requests?

My challenge to deflated leaders is to ask yourself 'Is part of the cause my lack of communication of the fact that I need to be treated as a human-being to these unthinking (not unkind) colleagues?'. Is their behaviour coming from a place of unkindness or from a place of unthinking? My guess is that it's the latter.

So, empathy teaches us to see that our leaders just have no clue about how they are making us feel. How could they know if we don't communicate this with compassion? Often we choose to believe they are invincible, right? They don't have a life outside work. They have no needs, no ups and downs. They are always available for us to message, grab for a moment, solve problems.

Isn't that how pet owners view us as vets and nurses? The pressure we feel because pet owners don't think about us as humans, wives, husbands, parents, pet owners ourselves is often raised as a concern. I understand why pet owners forget these things and it doesn't come from a place of unkindness. They just forget.

So, if clients forget that vets and nurses are human, it stands to reason that vets and nurses forget that head nurses, head vets and line managers are human. The chain continues up to the very top.

Do you ever imagine that your line manager is treated this way? Do you reckon the line managers treat their line managers in a similar way too?

Motivation

What do I want out of a situation and how do I achieve that?

Not surprisingly, many vets and nurse managers have low assertiveness and low self-esteem. We don't rock the boat, cause drama or make a fuss. We power on through.

I propose a healthier way to work. By pointing out how the team can better support each other, we can pave the way for real change in our professions.

The current 42% of vets and nurses seriously thinking about leaving the profession is unsustainable and more than disappointing. So, to the leaders who are used, treated like androids and never asked how their day is going, if you communicate with your good cognitive empathy and social skills to those around you that you are human too and need some empathy back, you are being truly kind to those who will learn these vital skills from you, and being a leader to the professions as a whole.

If one of us, as a leader, states the obvious, i.e. 'I am human, please treat me with compassion, empathy and like I'm more than just a vet or nurse or your manager', then that is an act of kindness which will have some long-lasting beneficial effects on our practices and on our lives.

We have to do something to change the 'norms' of our professions. Not starting isn't an option.

> *If you think you are too small to make a difference, try sleeping with a mosquito.*
>
> Dalai Lama

Social Media and Doom Surfing

- How do I stop doom surfing?

> The more negative a statement, the more likely we are to perceive it as truthful.

The human brain has evolved to detect change so when things turn out differently from what we'd hoped, we can easily start to dwell on the negative. In this manner, the brain has a negativity bias. Allowing our negativity bias to determine how we behave can have catastrophic effects on our mental wellbeing.

It's so easy for us to get overly focused on gathering information to support our survival, especially as external events on our news app exacerbate this inherent need. The key word here is 'overly'. The amount of time and effort we put into gathering this information is entirely within our control, and therefore so also are the personal effects of this information gathering.

Our social media 'survival' is also as important or as unimportant as we choose it to be. And if we allow it to consume us, we run the real danger of slipping into narcissistic behaviours which are widely known to cause mental health chaos.

The narcissist is obsessed with their image on social media as well as elsewhere. They crave 'likes' and re-tweets of their messages. They update their profile photo obsessively. Any time they are doing something admirable, a selfie has to be uploaded as a matter of importance. It is a lonely place to be, no matter how positive the feedback. Virtual positive acclaim does not bring the degree of contentment that the narcissist needs.

The human brain didn't really evolve to keep us happy, it evolved to keep us alive. And what kept us alive was the ability to be hypersensitive to problems and threats, such as predatory animals or harsh weather. Today, our challenges are much less severe but for all our wonderful evolutionary adaptations, our brain and nervous system don't really know that. The brain treats a stressful situation at work in the same way it

Mental Wellbeing and Positive Psychology for Veterinary Professionals: A Pre-emptive, Proactive and Solution-based Approach, First Edition. Laura Woodward.
© 2024 John Wiley & Sons Ltd. Published 2024 by John Wiley & Sons Ltd.

would treat an encounter with an approaching wild animal (although for us as veterinary professionals, the overlap can sometimes occur!).

After the stressful event, it replays the situation over and over, so we never forget about it. That's a really helpful thing if we spend our days out in the wilderness, but not so much when we're in the practice all day not surrounded by predators.

Research by Dr Richard Davidson (Davidson 2012) shows that the more negative a statement, the more likely we are to perceive it as truthful, given our tendency to pay more attention to the negative. In his publication 'Good things don't come easy (to mind)', he shows that 'The general phenomenon of a positive–negative asymmetry was extended to judgements of truth. That is, *negatively framed statements were shown to receive substantially higher truth ratings than equivalent statements framed positively.* However, the cognitive mechanisms underlying this effect are unknown, so far' (emphasis added).

So how often do you reach for the news feed on your phone each day? Maybe count the number of times per day you clock into your news app when you have a day off.

Why do you quickly check the headlines so many times each day? Many of my clients say it's because they are desperate for that one headline which will bring a positive, uplifting message. Just a bit of hope. And the sooner they read it, the sooner they will feel better. And that makes perfect sense.

During the COVID-19 pandemic, when news that the new Pfizer vaccine was 95% effective came out, a brief survey of 40 UK veterinarians in therapy indicated that a whopping 85% of them felt their mood lift that day, for the whole day (Laura Woodward Counselling 2020). This was soon followed by news of the new variant, cancelled Christmas and rising deaths, and their mood instantly reverted to sadness, fear and anxiety.

Others say they reach for their phone because they want to see the latest meme or TikTok for a brief minute of respite from reality. It brings joy which we can instantly share. I love spreading this instant joy. Also, because it's so brief and fleeting, we can use it as an exercise in *not* swiping from WhatsApp shared jokes or TikTok uploads to news headlines. It's as simple as making the conscious decision to not swipe.

So see how many times during the day you reach for your phone. Pause before you reach for it, take a breath and briefly ask yourself what you hope to achieve with this. It may be quickly checking whether you need to attend to a message/email. It may be an autopilot move you do whenever there is a pause in your hectic day or a ping.

Could you do something else for novelty's sake a few times instead, for example a mini-meditation or noticing what's gone right so far today?

Many therapists recommend checking your news feed a maximum of twice a day. If something major happens, that headline will stay. You won't miss it because you delayed checking your phone. Statistically, the chances of the latest headline being uplifting as opposed to upsetting are slim.

How Do I Stop Doom Surfing?

- *Reduce access*: turn off news notifications. There is no reason to get a news alert six times a day, and certainly no need to stay updated during the night – the news will still be there in the morning.
- *Screen time limits* aren't just for children. You can set limits for your own personal phone use. It's nearly impossible to estimate your daily screen time accurately by guessing. Taking control in order to be self-compassionate is a positive move.
- *Make it less entertaining:* another way to trick your brain. Make it less fun by shifting your phone to grayscale. You're basically removing some of the incentive for your brain to continue to scroll when you make it more boring.
- *Have a non-screen reading item* at the ready for bedtime and for those times when you do wake up in the middle of the night. My all-time favourite is 'Daily Doses of Wisdom' edited by Josh Bartok, a paperback with a thought-provoking snippet of wisdom on each page.
- *Flip the narrative and show some gratitude*: can you really express gratitude when you're stressed and agitated due to insomnia? Or at any time of the day? Make a conscious decision, instead of checking the news, to send a (potentially delayed) email or text of appreciation to someone.
- *Click-bait*: don't take the bait. Have self-control.
- *When you're with a friend*: what a compliment to leave your phone switched off or at least out of sight, and your kind, full attention on your friend.
- *Decide how much you want to read the news*, check Facebook and scroll through Twitter. Then decide how you are going to control

yourself and achieve this goal. One client of mine recently had trouble avoiding social media postings even though she really wanted to. She even deleted Instagram from her phone. But when the craving for an Insta hit got hold of her, she would just reinstall the app. We came up with a plan: every time she felt a craving for her next fix, she would turn her phone off completely and apply the oiliest hand cream she could find. Then she would massage her hands and breathe. It worked and she is no longer a social media junkie.

- Notice every time you consciously put this plan into action. Remind yourself why you're doing this. It may be to decrease stress or to be more present with your surroundings or friends. It's self-compassionate and kind.

When you feel yourself reaching for your phone because you have an urge to read the news, decide how to postpone that 'fix'. Pause. Take 10 mindful breaths. Ask yourself if you can skip this catch-up, i.e. take control in a self-compassionate way so that each and every time you unlock your phone, you're doing it mindfully rather than mindlessly. Every time you don't unlock your phone is a win over doom surfing.

Some people find it empowering to turn their phone off or leave it in another room for a few hours a day. They are in control of their phone rather than the other way around. However, that's unthinkable for others.

The world isn't all rainbows and lollipops. Getting control of your doom scrolling does not mean ignoring the real issues that exist. But if you find yourself seeking out more and more negative stories, your brain may be hooked and it's time to take it back.

So, the next time you 'need' to look at your phone, be self-compassionate and in control rather than on autopilot.

My son, there is a battle between two wolves inside of us all.
One is Evil: it is anger, jealousy and greed, resentment, lies and ego.
The other is Good: it is peace, love, kindness and empathy.
The boy asked 'Mum, which wolf wins?'.
The mother replied 'Why son, the one you feed, of course'.
Adapted from a Native American parable

References

Davidson, R. (2012). Good things don't come easy (to mind). Explaining framing effects in judgments of truth. *Experimental Psychology* 59: 38–46.

Laura Woodward Counselling. Survey Monkey survey 2020.

Yearning, Striving and Wishing Things Were Different

- 'Letting go' of striving
- What is striving?
- Blissful happiness

'Letting Go' of Striving

Shakespeare once said, 'Expectation is the root of all heartache'. By striving for someone or something to come and make us happy, we are inevitably saying to ourselves that until that person/thing/state of mind arrives, we are going to remain unfulfilled, unsatiated, incomplete.

Our greatest pains and disappointments arise from those things we try so hard to grasp and secure. We are constantly struggling to achieve and possess, or to feel 'things' which we don't yet feel.

Ironically, those very things we want, or *think* we want, often don't even exist or, if they do exist, rarely satisfy according to our illusions.

We live with a rampant imagination running wild and dictating our thirsty cravings. You drop your phone in the toilet but despite plunging it into a bucket of rice, it's damaged beyond repair. Yet you can't replace 'like with like'. Apple, Samsung, Blackberry, whoever, insists you have an upgrade to satisfy your ever-increasing needs, needs you didn't even know you had, thus further encouraging your desires to have more apps, better camera, faster downloads.

What is Striving?

Striving is *not* aiming to achieve a goal or a good intention. That's commendable. Striving is an unsatiated and insatiable yearning which doesn't leave us.

When we reach the place where we can let go of striving, we are liberated from the exhausting pursuit of chasing happiness.

Chögyam Trungpa Rinpoche said, 'There is no need to struggle to be free; the absence of struggle is in itself freedom'.

Mental Wellbeing and Positive Psychology for Veterinary Professionals: A Pre-emptive, Proactive and Solution-based Approach, First Edition. Laura Woodward.
© 2024 John Wiley & Sons Ltd. Published 2024 by John Wiley & Sons Ltd.

Before we learn to let go of striving, we will experience disappointments. Given the convoluted nature of desire, there are no experiences that are entirely free of disappointment. This is what makes disappointment such a complex and confusing feeling. Many of the desires that we pursue are unconscious, sublimated and frequently contradictory.

Paradoxically, we may even become disappointed when we get what we want. For example, in Sigmund Freud's 1916 essay 'Some Character-Types Met with in Psycho-Analytic Work', he explored the paradox of people who were 'wrecked by success'. Unconsciously, these people believed that their success was unjustified, so achieving it didn't feel satisfying to them.

In Chapter 5 of this section, I wrote about imposter syndrome. First described by psychologist Suzanne Imes, PhD, in the 1970s, Imposter syndrome occurs amongst high achievers who are unable to internalise and accept their success. They feel that they are a fraud and about to be 'found out' instead of being able to celebrate their well-earned successes big and small. In essence, they strived, they achieved and they were left anxious and empty.

It must be bewildering: to work so hard to get to where we want to be, only to find that we're still not happy or even cheerful. Even when we do get what we want – and think we deserve – we may discover that what we wanted so badly doesn't bring the bliss and happiness we expected.

So we may be striving to become head nurse in a busy practice or to be head surgeon in a referral institution or to manage our own branch in a corporate, but be careful what you wish for, and try not to rely on it as your only true chance of happiness or fulfilment. You may get there. You may believe you deserve it. Enjoy it for what it is without putting yourself under pressure to be blissfully happy and complete.

How do we 'let go' of striving? Jon Kabat-Zinn tells of a cruel practice in India, where there is a method of catching monkeys that involves cutting a small hole in the top of a coconut, then attaching the coconut by a wire to the base of a tree. A banana is put inside the coconut. When a monkey slides its hand in to get the banana and holds onto it, its closed fist is too big to slide back out. The monkey becomes trapped as it does not want to let go. And yet if the monkey let go of the banana, it could easily remove its hand and be free.

During mindful meditation, we can decide to 'let go' of striving for the perfect life/thing/person. By accepting what we already have as good enough, we can be liberated from the entrapment and the nagging need for more and more and more.

We don't have to stop improving ourselves or our talents. We don't have to cancel all CPD or social engagements. It's about accepting ourselves as we are, while enjoying the journey of self-improvement. It's about noticing what's good about something, someone, some feeling, without worrying about what's not perfect about it.

Then, like a butterfly, just when you're least expecting it, happiness and completeness may land on your shoulder.

Blissful Happiness

If we can let go of striving for something which constantly eludes us (blissful happiness), then we can be so much more free of angst than we are now.

Happiness is like a butterfly:

> *The more you chase it, the more it will elude you.*
> *But if you turn your attention to other things,*
> *it will come and sit softly on your shoulder*
>
> Henry David Thoreau

It is both human nature and culturally instilled behaviour to seek lasting security, happiness and transcendent meaning amidst the roller-coaster ride of fleeting conditions: lots of beer followed by the mother of all hangovers, financial gains followed by losses, approval one day, criticism the next, four great fracture repairs followed by one depressing wound breakdown. In hunting down and latching onto what feels great, we inevitably experience the disappointment that arises when something is only just about good enough.

We work, we earn, we spend and yet, we are left feeling empty. Despite the retail therapy, we think, 'I'm still not everlastingly happy. Am I missing something here?'.

What about all those people out there living in their airy, open-plan, tidy homes with vast glass doors and well-behaved children? How do they never experience sadness, depression or fear? If only we could find the perfect job to buy a large new house with spectacular river views, wardrobes wedged with fabulous clothes, our dinner parties would attract all the right people. And then, as sophisticated friends laughed at our jokes and never tired of offering admiration, we'd finally be inoculated from pain and everything would turn out just perfect.

And so, the relaxation and satisfaction we seek are always somewhere down the line, and we believe that this moment now is incapable of providing us with anything worthwhile. If we can get through this moment, then that moment, surely some moment sometime will be a suitable one in which to stop striving and to enjoy life.

The paradox of hedonism, also called the pleasure paradox, refers to the practical difficulties encountered in the pursuit of pleasure. For the hedonist, constant pleasure seeking may not yield the most actual pleasure or happiness in the long term, or short term, when consciously pursuing pleasure interferes with experiencing it.

(From Wikipedia)

One doesn't need to be a psychologist to know that constant busyness is a symptom of avoidance. When we run out of fuel and idle to a full stop, what do we experience? The voidness of meaning that is simply surviving in this world. When unfulfilled or sad, we power on through. There's plenty to keep us busy as vets, nurses and managers.

Meanwhile, until that elusive moment arrives, we keep ourselves busy. If being insanely busy at work brings you pleasure, you're probably in the right job. If work is slow and boring, it often brings the team down despite the chance to rest.

I could do so much more in my chasing of happiness if only my phone didn't keep hopping, reminding me that I am in contact with my friends. And yet, it's hiding in plain sight that having friends message me could bring me enough joy that I could stop running after the dream of pure bliss.

And when we are physically with a friend, how many of us interrupt our conversation to glance at our smart watch, checking in on who has just connected with us? Do we switch off from the conversation when we hear a ping? So, the value we put on our friendships is measured in numbers of friends and not in the quality of the face-to-face time we have with them.

Maybe, if our friends can't fulfil our emotional needs, we can book a hike in the Himalayas, traverse the Andes or go spelunking Mexico's caves. And maybe, just maybe, we will find the life satisfaction we crave there.

While new experiences have their place, they provide as much lasting inner peace as impulsive sex with multiple partners provides true intimacy. Thrills are a lot of fun, holidays in Iceland are truly awesome, they add spice to life, but we're in for a big let-down if this is where we're to find lifelong serenity.

And that is where the secret lies. If we can be with this moment and really present, maybe it can be 'good enough'. If we can let go of striving for something which constantly eludes us (blissful happiness), then we can be so much more free of angst than we are now.

Otherwise we are just chasing ends of rainbows which move farther and farther away the closer we get to them.

The key to these refuges lies in understanding one simple but profound truth: what really matters in life is how we react to situations and circumstances, rather than the situations and circumstances themselves.

Our present attitudes produce our future perspectives. So, we *can* be happy on our own Ikea sofa without the river view. It's a choice. We can meet up with one friend and immerse ourselves in their company, savouring the conversation with our phone elsewhere and at another time.

And if you are lucky enough to be backpacking in Thailand, camping in the wilderness or hiking to the top of Kilimanjaro, you can be totally and completely present in the moment while not taking selfies, updating your status on Facebook or filming for your YouTube channel.

The more you are present and mindfully observing the view in Iceland, the longer the beautiful effects of awe will bring you joy. These moments when you just look are moments when it is so easy to learn how to be present. It's stunning. Recording it will be great for the future. Photography is an act of mindfulness in itself. Just let's not forget to absorb the beauty while we're actually there.

Only by being truly present in the moment can we choose to be satisfied with it. We can literally choose to be completely satisfied. What better way to foster an unflappable psyche?

Moral Injury

- What can we do about moral injury?
- Moral courage

When something goes wrong at work, it hurts and damages our core. The workplace insists we move on, but this incident can become a demon which keeps raising its ugly head if we don't face it.

Moral injury also happens when we are pressured into overworking cases for financial gain or when we feel we are charging too much for services. If the pet owner chooses a cheaper alternative treatment to what we recommend or, worse, chooses no treatment all due to the cost, we are left knowing that we could have done better for that patient.

Moral injury can leave us with long-term psychological scars if we allow it to. The feeling that we cannot perform as well as we should, and that our patients and clients will inevitably suffer, is hard to come to terms with. It happens in every practice from the most expensive hospitals in London to the charities all over the country and even in charities treating stray dogs in India for nothing.

During the COVID-19 pandemic, we handed our ventilators over to the NHS. Whether you think that's morally right or wrong, it followed that some of our patients may have died as a result and we wouldn't be able to feel that we did everything we could do for them.

These 'moral injuries', injuries to our ethics, can have long-lasting negative psychological effects. Sir Simon Wessely, professor of psychological medicine at the Institute of Psychiatry, King's College London, defines moral injury as 'where you know you didn't do everything you could have done'. It makes us feel angry, it makes us feel guilty and it makes us feel ashamed.

In a highly regarded tier 3 hospital in London, a vet nervously makes the call to an owner to advise them of further investigations and treatment their dog needs. The prognosis is guarded, the injuries are life changing, the owner is devoted to their pet, the dog is wonderful and young.

What's the most difficult part of the conversation? Is it the part about describing the injuries? Is it explaining in layperson's terms what the

Mental Wellbeing and Positive Psychology for Veterinary Professionals: A Pre-emptive, Proactive and Solution-based Approach, First Edition. Laura Woodward.
© 2024 John Wiley & Sons Ltd. Published 2024 by John Wiley & Sons Ltd.

treatment entails? No. It's giving the estimate of costs to the owner. A cost the vet already feels is extortionate even though they know the treatment is the gold standard.

There is anxiety that the owner will say that's too much, they can't pay that or they will go somewhere else where maybe the expertise isn't as high.

The call about the guarded prognosis, the life-changing injuries, the tragedy of it all is something we're used to. It's sad but it's easier when it's not your own pet. But giving an enormous estimate, even if you can get the words out, and waiting for the gasp at the other end of the phone is horrible. Then there's the lengthy wait while that owner has to go consult with the other owner and you know there will be another gasp of horror at the costs. You have to wait, sitting with anxiety and all the precursors to moral injury building up within you.

If the client agrees, the treatment goes according to plan, the dog does well and the client pays the bill, we can move on. But if they choose the cheaper alternative, or substandard treatment, or if they go elsewhere and you can't bring yourself to follow it up, it adds to the pile of moral injuries sitting within us and the guilt and shame grow subconsciously.

Imagine you're a nurse in a busy charity. Pets pile in to be neutered or vaccinated for minimal cost and that's a great feeling of getting through a long ops list. Others pile in from expensive private practices and you can care for them effectively because the clients make an audible sigh of relief when you tell them how much you'd like them to pay for a procedure like a cystotomy or foreign body removal.

But you also have patients who need a full work-up and expensive treatments. Full bloods, ultrasound and three days hospitalisation for a simple pancreatitis. You don't have the funds. You have to choose who gets the kennel and what drugs you can and can't give because they cost too much even though it's clear what this patient needs to make a great, swift recovery with an excellent prognosis. Your hands are tied. You send them home with substandard treatment which will probably work although it will take longer and the dog will feel rubbish for days more than he would have if he had wealthy owners.

Then there are the owners who might have been waiting weeks for their 10-minute consultation with you. By this time, many have thought of a shopping list of their pet's issues because they care and they love their pet. It's coming into a charity vaccination clinic, but it has skin, ear and teeth issues.

The owner adores their pet and some of our lonelier pet owners might have spent all morning getting ready for this golden opportunity to go to the clinic and get everything sorted, including having a bit of human company.

We have to do what we can with the resources we have. It's a rush to examine the pet, listen to the owner and interact with them because it's clear they are asking for our company too. We prescribe what we have on the shelf which isn't always as effective as what we want to prescribe, then we send the owner and pet out the door knowing that we could have done better and been kinder.

Yes, we're doing a wonderful job and the charities are a god-send for people who can't afford private vet bills. Because of the charities, many people can have the company of a cat or dog instead of it being a privilege of the wealthy. But for us, it often doesn't sit right. Yes, we become immune to it with time. Or we think we're immune.

In a busy NHS hospital, rounds take place in the acute medicine department to decide who gets the remaining ICU beds and who doesn't. It may even be a life-or-death decision. Even their hands are tied. Specialists try to be logical and unemotional, nearly mathematical about these decisions and they do a great job of keeping emotions out of the field. But all the while, moral injury can be building up inside us.

The stray dogs in India are gorgeous. Where I worked, in Visakhapatnam, they hung around in groups, pecking order all sorted out without the need for human intervention. Local people fed them scraps and they got more from the bins. In some places they were a bit fat. They were calm, friendly and happy. But if they needed anything more than neutering and vaccination, my hands were tied. I couldn't do anything for the sick ones or the fractured ones apart from look away. It still pains me years on.

What Can We Do About Moral Injury?

In the *European Journal of Psychotraumatology*, Siobhan Hegarty defines moral injury (Hegarty et al. 2022):

> Moral injury: the strong emotional and cognitive reactions following events which clash with someone's moral code, values or expectations.

The healthcare workers in this article expressed their increased anxiety, depression and sleep disturbances due to moral injury during the COVID-19 pandemic.

In the *BMC of Psychiatry*, Amsalem et al. (2021) described 72% of the healthcare workers in the study reporting moral injury causing anxiety, depression and/or PTSD disorders at baseline during the COVID era, 62% at day 30 and 64% at day 90. Disorders also included suicidal ideation (Amsalem et al. 2021).

The injury doesn't fade after a glass of wine and a good night's sleep.

In *Medsurg Nursing*, Vicki Lachman (2016) talks about moral resilience as the buffer between moral injury and the long-term pathopsychological effects it can cause.

> *Moral resilience is the ability to deal with an ethically adverse situation without lasting effects of moral distress and moral residue.*
> Vicki Lachman (2016)

Moral resilience is something we should aim to develop *prior to* morally injurious events (MIEs). Another argument for giving this book and other support to our students, student nurses and new grads.

Morally resilient vets and nurses have already learnt emotional intelligence prior to MIEs. They have the ability to see an MIE, notice the immediate effects of real-time moral injury and its potential for long-term effects on them. They are self-aware and through this awareness and by practising self-regulation can avoid ruminating and the self-flagellation which can ensue.

Sometimes, we have to be as mathematical as the hospital managers who decide who gets the ICU bed, and to forgive ourselves for having to make these decisions (see Part Six, Chapter 11 on compassion).

Moral Courage

Moral courage is necessary to accept that we will face many of these scenarios at work and will have to make difficult decisions against our better clinical judgement. We can prepare ourselves for this prior to the events.

Moral courage and moral resilience don't negate the pain we feel when we provide substandard care against our will. By allowing the pain to be present, by facing it while doing the best we can with the resources we have, we can be morally injured and then recover from that injury and go on to provide good care without experiencing depression, PTSD and other pathopsychological long-term effects.

References

Amsalem, D., Lazarov, A., Markowitz, J.C. et al. (2021). Psychiatric symptoms and moral injury among US healthcare workers in the COVID-19 era. *BMC Psychiatry* 21 (1): 546.

Hegarty, S., Lamb, D., Stevelink, S.A.M. et al. (2022). 'It hurts your heart': frontline healthcare worker experiences of moral injury during the COVID-19 pandemic. *European Journal of Psychotraumatology* 13 (2): 2128028.

Lachman, V.D. (2016). Moral resilience: managing and preventing moral distress and moral residue. *Medsurg Nursing* 25 (2): 121–124.

Identity

- When being a veterinary professional is your whole identity
- How did we get to this situation?
- How do you know if your identity has become enmeshed with your career?
- Start small

There's more to us than our labels. Often, our professions are so interesting to others that our identity gets lost. When being a vet or a vet nurse is your whole identity, it can reduce your life as a whole human being to just a concept.

While identifying closely with your career isn't necessarily bad, it makes you vulnerable to a painful identity crisis if you choose to change career paths, work part time or even burn out.

When Being a Veterinary Professional is Your Whole Identity

Psychologists use the term 'enmeshment' to describe the situation when boundaries between people become blurred and individual identities become unimportant, eroding one's sense of self.

Many vets and nurses I counsel have become enmeshed not with their partners but with their careers. 'What am I, if not a vet or vet nurse?'

You know how it is. You're introduced as 'X the vet nurse' or as 'Y the vet'. It's an immediate icebreaker. We're so easy to talk to because we're full of stories about the most unusual type of animal we've ever treated, etc.

> A particular confluence of high achievement, intense competitiveness and culture of overwork has caught many in a perfect storm of career enmeshment and burnout.

Over the years, we've found that these issues interact in such complex ways with people's identity, personality and emotions that it often requires full-on psychological therapy to address them successfully.

Mental Wellbeing and Positive Psychology for Veterinary Professionals: A Pre-emptive, Proactive and Solution-based Approach, First Edition. Laura Woodward.
© 2024 John Wiley & Sons Ltd. Published 2024 by John Wiley & Sons Ltd.

How Did We Get to This Situation?

A culture where staying behind after work late into the night is considered the norm, and leaving on time is a bit weird, doesn't help us to have a life outside work where we can exercise our non-veterinary identity.

Maybe our job is all that we see of value in ourselves. This belief is further cemented by our families who are so proud we graduated and by strangers at dinner parties who are in awe of how interesting our jobs are.

But constructing one's identity around a career is a risky move although it may feel very comfortable for very many years. What if you get the sack, particularly from a big corporation, making it especially difficult to get another post? What if you become disabled or unable to continue your specialisation due to physical problems? What if you need to move geographically and you're middle aged? Who wants an expensive middle-aged vet or nurse when we can have such good new grads?

No matter how it happens, becoming disconnected from a career that forms the foundation of your identity can lead to bigger issues, such as depression, anxiety, substance misuse and loneliness

How Do You Know if Your Identity Has Become Enmeshed with Your Career?

Ask yourself the following questions.

- How often do you think about work when you're not at work?
- How do you describe yourself on Tinder?
- How long after you've just met someone do they know what you do for a living?
- Where do you spend most of your time?

If you are concerned that you are unhealthily enmeshed with being a vet or vet nurse, maybe try to extend yourself out of that enmeshment, although it takes some bravery.

Start Small

You don't need to run a marathon to get exercise. Maybe just walk and run without having to achieve anything. We've been high achievers ever since the 11-plus exams. Give it a rest. Running and walking mindfully vastly increase their emotional benefits. Run and walk fast for exercise. Maybe do both.

The important concept is to notice that you can do an activity without achieving any points, steps, goals, postnominals. Try giving achieving a rest.

In his book *Friends: Understanding the Power of Our Most Important Relationships*, Robin Dunbar showed that the optimum number of close friends associated with good mental health was 3–5. Reaching out to 3–5 friends who are not veterinary based can help us to become a bit less enmeshed with the job.

We all know the narcissists out there who crave attention and reaffirmation, who are out canvassing for popularity six nights a week desperate for the masses to adore them and boost their sense of self. The people who send a party invite to 110 of their closest friends on WhatsApp so everyone can see how many friends they have. This is a concerning sign of poor mental health.

So, reconnect for sure but again, like not running a marathon, we don't have to build up an impressive portfolio of friends in a competitive fashion just to clock up the numbers.

Look beyond your job title. Consider reframing your relationship with your career not simply in terms of your company or title, but in terms of your skills that could be used across different contexts. For example, many psychotherapists who burn out find that their skills translate well to human resources management or guidance counselling.

While identifying closely with your career isn't necessarily bad, it makes you vulnerable to a painful identity crisis if you burn out, get laid off or retire. Individuals in these situations frequently suffer anxiety, depression and despair. By claiming back some time for yourself and diversifying your activities and relationships, you can build a more balanced and robust identity in line with your values.

Bullying

- Cancel culture
- How to refrain from punitive actions

In 2021, the Mind Matters Initiative in the UK ran a survey amongst student vet nurses, recent grad vet nurses and clinical coaches in UK practices (vetmindmatters.org). Over 650 people responded, 96% of whom agreed or strongly agreed that bullying and incivility were serious problems in the veterinary professions.

In this MMI survey, only 18% said they believed that veterinary nursing is a well-respected profession. Many vets still aren't aware that veterinary nursing *is* a profession formally recognised in law since 1991.

Twenty percent of respondents had witnessed or experienced discrimination in their practice. It's hard to comprehend how discrimination can be so common in this day and age. Being discriminatory is not cool and neither is it productive, authoritarian or even acceptable.

What *is* helpful, respectable and necessary as a matter of urgency is for all of us to have the courage to call out this outdated, damaging behaviour and address it in the open.

I once worked with a tremendously clever vet. They were an expert in their field. They knew everything in the literature and beyond. A fantastic colleague in that regard. However, this colleague felt it was completely okay to shout at team members for being imperfect. People might be in tears, confidence in tatters and productivity running at zero because of these tirades, and yet the shouting continued. They even once kicked a kennel door in anger even though there was a dog inside. There were 15 of us in the prep room when that happened. How many people called them out and put a stop to the repeated behaviours? One.

Mental Wellbeing and Positive Psychology for Veterinary Professionals: A Pre-emptive, Proactive and Solution-based Approach, First Edition. Laura Woodward.
© 2024 John Wiley & Sons Ltd. Published 2024 by John Wiley & Sons Ltd.

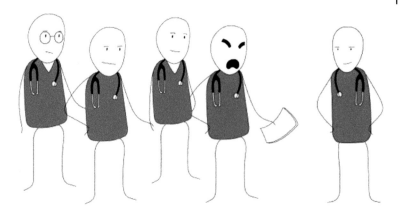

The question is why, when we know that this behaviour is completely unacceptable and damaging in many ways, we don't call it out and put a stop to it?

I've asked several colleagues about this. It seems that we are so afraid of becoming the next target of toxic abuse that we would rather allow abuse of our colleague to continue rather than become that target.

This is how people feel. We can scorn them for being weak, we can judge all the bystanders, or we can be the person who stands up to anyone exerting bullying or even unkind and unhelpful behaviours with the words 'We don't work like that here'. Or 'That behaviour is not acceptable in this team'. Anything you say will help, you just need to say it. It's as easy as speaking.

> If you see it, call it out: it's as simple as speaking.

Cancel Culture

In *Psychology Today*, Dr Utpal Dholakia talks about cancel culture.

> In this act of cancelling, the canceller calls out a real or perceived transgression by the cancelled entity (often a celebrity or an organisation).
>
> The canceller is outraged, disgusted and angry.
>
> Typically they call out the transgression through social media platforms seeking active retaliation by the masses towards the

cancelled entity. Visible social isolation, punishment and public shaming are victories for the canceller.

The difference between cancelling and calling out a specific behaviour when appropriate is that, to many observers, the canceller's actions often seem disproportionate to the magnitude of the transgression.

Why is this? Perhaps it's because the canceller is looking for an outlet for their rage. Perhaps because naming and shaming does actually work. Videoing atrocities and making them viral works.

Back to bullying in the workplace and calling it out. Whether we like it or not, there will be people we work with who are socially unskilled. There will be bullies, there will be people with low self-esteem, depression, anxiety and blissful happiness. From my experience of large workplaces, everyone has 'stuff' going on in their lives.

So calling out the bully is essential. Ghosting, cancelling or boycotting them is unproductive.

How to Refrain from Punitive Actions

Probably emotional intelligence is a good place to start.

- *Self-awareness*: what emotions does this person's actions bring up in you?
- *Self-regulation*: having made the space between their action and my reaction, what can I say or do to achieve the outcome I want (motivation)?
- *Motivation*: there is something to be gained if my reaction is appropriate and proportionate to the transgression.
- *Empathy*: there are multiple reasons behind this person's bullying actions. Rarely are serial bullies content, happy and at peace with life.
- *Social skills*: brave body language, courageous eye contact, carefully chosen words can put this episode to bed.

> If 96% of nurses say that bullying and incivility are serious problems in the veterinary workplace, we need to take action today.

Conflict and Client Complaints

Conflict is a normal part of being human. Conflict inside and outside of work is unavoidable.

> You can't change all the other people; you can only change your reaction to them.

Conflict can come at us from all directions and we may so easily cause conflict ourselves. There may be conflict between us and our partner, our parents, siblings, children, neighbours. We might have conflicting views with another driver about whether we, the cyclist, or they, the car driver, has the right of way.

We will discuss team conflict in the next chapter.

Conflict between us and the owners of the pets we cherish is painful. The client complaint letter is gut wrenching to receive. No matter how 'right' or 'wrong' the client is, it will affect us.

There will always be complaints whether we deserve them or not. We may receive chocolates and wine from the owners of a patient we euthanised with compassion and expertise and then be handed a complaint from a client whose pet received the very best of care and made a remarkable recovery.

Why?

There are a multitude of causes which we can change, as we know: better communication, accurate estimates being given, returning phone calls promptly, etc. Most practices aim to do all of these.

But what if we provided excellent care, top-class communication, accurate estimates and a fantastic outcome and still get a complaint?

We can bitch about the client, we can throw our hands in the air, we can ignore them. However, the effect remains. Our focus remains on the complaint rather than on anything else which happened that day.

Knowing in advance that this scenario is going to play out, what can we do to change our reaction to the people we can't change? I advocate using emotional intelligence in the management of conflict.

Mental Wellbeing and Positive Psychology for Veterinary Professionals: A Pre-emptive, Proactive and Solution-based Approach, First Edition. Laura Woodward.

Once you walk your way through the five competencies a few times during episodes of conflict, it becomes more natural and most people choose to adopt these methods as their regular response to conflict.

I once had a client with a small fluffy white dog which they presented to my colleague recumbent and screaming. After appropriate analgesia and investigations, we diagnosed cervical spinal compression involving two discs. The client understood, our communication was clear, I gave an accurate estimate, listed the potential complications and potential outcomes and she consented. She seemed unconcerned about the cost, which helped. She did tell me that the dog only ever ate off a white dinner plate and asked me to ensure that this message was passed onto whoever would be feeding her. I did that.

I did the appropriate surgery and over the following week the dog made an uneventful recovery. 'Uneventful' doesn't describe the hours of physio, the hand feeding of her full resting energy requirement (RER), the back-breaking support of her as she toddled about the physio room, the insomnia and then the wonderful, celebratory feeling we felt during that week as she progressed. It was a fantastic week for our team.

She was discharged to the owner who seemed to have forgotten the chocolates and thank-you card.

A week later, I received a formal complaint from the owner. Whilst she appreciated that we had fulfilled our obligations and cured her dog, she was desperately upset that I had not made sure that the dog was fed off a white dinner plate.

I was aghast. The ward nurses had indeed fed this gorgeous dog from a white dinner plate five times a day and she was taking in her carefully calculated RER every day.

When I spoke to the owner, ready to defend myself and my team with eloquence and power, she said that anyone would know that she meant a porcelain dinner plate and not a plastic one. I soon realised that the chocolates and card were not coming my way.

I confess that I threw my hands in the air and complained loudly about this owner. Did that relieve my angst? Not a bit. Because you cannot change other people, you can only change your reaction to them.

My reaction to this lady was judgemental (she was 'wrong'), lacking in empathy (I cannot relate to her distress), angry, defensive and dismissive.

After some thought and contemplation, I decided to put emotional intelligence into the mix and see if I could get rid of this horrible feeling.

Self-awareness: I feel wronged, unappreciated, angry, sad, resentful.

Self-regulation: I want to bitch, moan and point out to her in a massive email just how wrong she is. However, I choose not to.

> Between action and reaction there is a space. In that space we have the power to choose our reaction.

I phoned the owner to see if she would come into the practice, without her dog, for a face-to-face chat. She did.

Motivation: what do I want out of this situation and how can I achieve that? Well, to be honest, I want this person to change. I want her to appreciate all the intricacies of discectomies and ventral slots and tell me how wonderful we all are. I want the chocolates and the thank-you card.

Empathy: this is where it gets hard. I found it so difficult to see things from her perspective. And that's the case for so many of the complaints we receive. We cannot relate to their grievances. Without being able to see things from their perspective, it's impossible to truly move on.

> Empathy means seeing something from someone else's perspective. It doesn't mean we have to agree with them. That's the key.

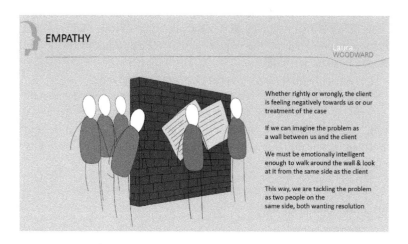

EMPATHY

Laura WOODWARD

Whether rightly or wrongly, the client is feeling negatively towards us or our treatment of the case

If we can imagine the problem as a wall between us and the client

We must be emotionally intelligent enough to walk around the wall & look at it from the same side as the client

This way, we are tackling the problem as two people on the same side, both wanting resolution

I forced myself to see it from her perspective. She had explicitly told me that her dog only ever ate off a white dinner plate. She was more adamant about that than she was about anything else at a time when I would have been focusing on my dog's spinal cord.

She, rightly or wrongly, presumed that I would know that that, of course, meant porcelain. Because, honestly, how many people eat off white melamine dinner plates unless they're camping?

She felt aggrieved that I hadn't listened to her (even though I had). She felt unappreciated, ignored and belittled by our lack of taking her seriously.

Social skills: we sat in the consult room on two chairs at a slight angle to each other.

Instead of painstakingly pointing out to her how wonderful we were and how wrong she was, I told her that I appreciated now that of course she meant a porcelain plate; and that she presumed that I would know that.

I didn't accuse her of making unfounded presumptions. I told her that I could see that it looked to her as though we didn't care as much as she needed us to care.

I could also understand that if you don't see with your own eyes how much time, effort and care we lavish on our patients, you just cannot appreciate it as much as we, the team, do.

At no stage did I apologise or defend. I just saw it from her side and verbalised that directly to her.

She didn't want an apology. She already thought we were highly skilled and worth every penny. She was delighted with her dog's recovery. She needed to be understood.

The chocolates and thank-you card arrived the next day.

Whether you would have reacted differently or not is fine. If someone feels this is inappropriate, that's okay. However, for us as a team, we were able to go back to the group celebratory mood with pride and chocolate and I use this emotionally intelligent approach with pretty much any conflict I experience as a life choice.

> Self-control is strength.
> Right thought is mastery.
> Calmness is power.

Team Dynamics

- Team dynamics and difficult colleagues
- Team dynamics and helping colleagues

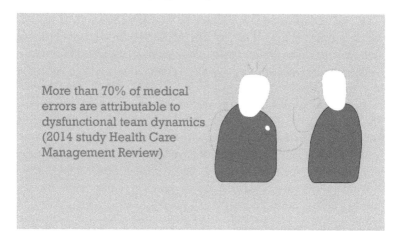

More than 70% of medical errors are attributable to dysfunctional team dynamics (2014 study Health Care Management Review)

Team Dynamics and Difficult Colleagues

We all want to work in a cohesive team with minimal conflict and stress. Whether it's because of the above statistic or otherwise, as managers, we relish when the team are getting on well and feel nauseous when there is bullying and hierarchy battles. It saps the strength of all team members when there is apparent favouritism or lack of tolerance or, dare I say it, even prejudice present in the practice.

Parable of the Good Samaritan

In the parable of the Good Samaritan, Jesus used the example of the Jew and the Samaritan, who would not ordinarily have been friendly towards each other. However, out of all of those who could have helped the Jew, only the Samaritan did.

Jesus tells of a man who was travelling from Jerusalem to Jericho and was attacked by robbers on the way. He was badly beaten and left for dead.

The first person to pass the injured man was a priest, who crossed the road away from him and continued walking.

The second person to pass the injured man was a Levite, a priest's assistant. He also crossed the road and continued walking without helping the man.

The third person to come by was a Samaritan, a person from Samaria. The Samaritans were hated by the Jews.

When the Samaritan saw the man, he took pity on him. He cleaned his wounds and bandaged him. He then put him on the back of his donkey and took him to an innkeeper, whom he paid to look after him.

The parable ends with Jesus giving a commandment to go out and do the same as the Samaritan had done.

This teaching of loving one's enemies is repeated in Matthew's Gospel, throughout many Buddhist texts, Islamic teachings, Hinduism and in other religions. How does this apply to us?

Well, as vets and nurses, we will have been exposed to a large cohort of personality types during our journey to this job. Possibly high achievers, many university students, lots of vets. Of course, we've met and been close to many other people. This is just a bit of a generalisation to explore.

As vet nurses, we will sometimes have been at university and sometimes been training in practice whilst at college. Often, new graduate vets are older than new graduate nurses. Often, experienced nurses are older than new graduate vets (and more highly skilled in some procedures). Yet both are integral to the job we do, and neither could do their job without the other.

We are bound together. Often, we are ensconced in the operating theatre for hours at a time together even if we don't really like each other.

There is a necessary hierarchy of new graduate to experienced nurse or vet, to head nurse or vet and all the clinical leads and deputy positions in between. We will be a mix of cultures, races, religions, genders and neurodiversities.

The link between the parable of the Good Samaritan and this is that we simply have to put our differences aside and get on in order to get the job done. Whether I like my team mate or not should never stop my working with them in a professional manner, whether I'm used to 'people like that' or not.

Loving one's enemies is something which is very hard and often impossible. However, professional tolerance is essential.

If we can push ourselves and our teams to go further and have empathy with one another no matter what, show kindness at all times especially when it's difficult to do so, and to be more than just tolerant of the difficult personalities in our colleagues, we will ultimately benefit in emotional and practical ways.

If I can be more aware of my colleagues' own struggles or at least that they may very well have some struggles, I may feel less alone in my own personal struggles.

If my colleagues are neurodiverse and trying to navigate a workplace which doesn't understand their needs, I can advocate for them and applaud their strength to be working in a largely neurotypical world.

Then maybe I will get the life satisfaction which the Good Samaritan inevitably had in ways I never dreamt possible before.

Team Dynamics and Helping Colleagues

A very important study done in 2015 at Princeton Theological Seminary (https://psycnet.apa.org/record/1973-31215-001) asks why it is that, when all of us have so many opportunities to help, we do sometimes and we don't at other times.

A group of divinity students at the Princeton Theological Seminary were told that they were going to give a practice sermon and they were each given a sermon topic. Half of the students were given the parable of the Good Samaritan (see above) and the other half were given random bible topics. Then, one by one, they were told they had to go to another building and give their sermon.

As they went from one building to the other, each of them passed an actor who was bent over and moaning, clearly in pain and in need.

Did they stop to help? The more interesting question is: Did it matter if they were contemplating the parable of the Good Samaritan or some other bible topic?

The answer is no, not at all. What turned out to be the deciding factors in whether they stopped to help a stranger in need or kept walking was how much of a hurry they thought they were in, and how much they were worried about giving their sermon.

I know for sure that I don't take every opportunity I have to help all others because my focus is elsewhere and I'm always in a hurry. I'm not alone in this predicament. In fact, what veterinary practice is so quiet that we can all take as much time as necessary to tend to the emotional needs of all our colleagues as well as our own needs?

The question is, when we do have the time, any time, are we then strong enough and willing enough to focus on others as well? Or are we so completely self-absorbed that we don't even notice their distress or difficulties?

Self-compassion and self-care are essential if we are to be of any help to others. We do need to start with ourselves before we give emotional strength to others. However, waiting for our lives to be perfect before we give anything isn't the aim.

> We can be self-compassionate at the same time as helping others. In fact, they are inextricably intertwined.

There is a relatively new field in brain studies called social neuroscience. This uses fMRI to look at the circuitry in two people's brains while they interact. The new thinking about compassion arising from social neuroscience is that our default wiring is to help. That is to say, if we attend to the other person, we automatically empathise, we automatically feel with them (emotional empathy). There are mirror neurons being activated in both brains in exactly the same areas. If that person is distressed, we are automatically prepared to help. The people who action that help are the empathically concerned people.

The question is: Why don't we help?

If we are preoccupied, we don't notice.

If we are self-absorbed, we don't notice.

If we are deep in social media, we don't notice.

If we don't notice, we can't have empathy and our mirror neurons are dormant.

Notice

So, in order to experience the joy and strength I can have as a strong practice member, in order to build a compassionate, tolerant, kind and bonded team, in order to avoid depersonalistion at work, when I have a moment free, it is very worthwhile to look around me, notice, take a breath and be grateful that we are a team of people, with all our foibles and diverse colourful backgrounds.

Compassion

If I can extend that noticing to feeling compassionate and wanting all of my colleagues to have a good day, that will make my day better. If my day is better, I have already improved the team dynamics and the standard of care of our patients.

Depression

Depression is a crippling cycle of self-fulfilling despair, where the sufferer often just can't see the exit point or, if they can see it, they can't get to it.

People with a family history of depression are more likely to experience depression themselves. In particular, maternal mental health difficulties can be a precursor.

There may be one trigger initially or there may be a combination of triggers and causes.

Maybe there's no obvious trigger or starting point. In any case, often identifying the starting point isn't necessary or even helpful to the person who is stuck.

Depression is common. At least 10% of us will experience it at some point. You are not alone.

People describe their depression as a darkness, emotional exhaustion, inability to even get out of the bed despite knowing that it has to be done.

For the onlooker, it may be hard to watch as they offer help and suggest things which they know will help others to feel good, such as a walk, company, doing something kind, listening to music.

But for the person who is truly depressed, despite knowing what may help, it's often literally physically impossible to put anything into action.

Depression is hopelessness, crying for no obvious reason, lack of motivation and sometimes anger that you're feeling this way. It is shame and guilt. Unaddressed, depression can lead to a lifetime of feeling just awful.

For managers and people who have never felt this way, it's important to note that when someone is depressed, they simply cannot phone that number on the poster you put up. It's beyond their ability to gather enough motivation to be proactive and ring it.

The NHS doesn't have the resources to help every depressed person, so waiting lists for therapy escalate to such a degree that, if you're lucky, a therapist will have a phone consultation with you in a few weeks' or months' time. GP's want you to have CBT and other therapies, but they know there may be a long wait.

Prescribing antidepressants after a phone consultation can be of real help to boost the sufferer and get them to a place where they gain some motivation to action some help.

Mental Wellbeing and Positive Psychology for Veterinary Professionals: A Pre-emptive, Proactive and Solution-based Approach, First Edition. Laura Woodward.
© 2024 John Wiley & Sons Ltd. Published 2024 by John Wiley & Sons Ltd.

Mindfulness, meditation and exercise are prescribed by the NHS to treat depression alongside medications and therapy.

If you are the sufferer, if you can just say it out loud, maybe your colleague or friend can help. If you were drowning, you would shout for help. Depression needs you to shout for help too. Crippling depression sometimes means you don't even have enough motivation to shout.

If you are the friend, colleague or manager who sees the signs of depression, you may feel helpless. And yet, just listening attentively, dropping everything to be inquisitive, not passing judgement or listing cures for depression might be the greatest help that person has ever had.

If you can follow that up, take action and book a consultation with their GP, an appointment with a mental health professional, or even both, you will be doing so much more than sticking a helpline poster up or just giving advice which they simply can't follow.

That is empathic concern and you, as the listener, are not alone either.

Anger

There's nothing 'wrong' about feeling angry. It's a powerful, colourful and often helpful emotion. It is what you choose to do with this emotion internally and externally which determines how it affects you and those around you.

> *Anyone can be angry - that is easy. But to be angry with the right person, to the right degree, at the right time, for the right purpose, and in the right way; this is not easy.*
>
> Aristotle

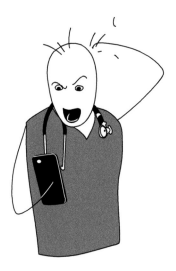

It's normal to get angry, right? Clients can be unreasonable, colleagues can be infuriating, family members can drive you to distraction and other road users are intolerable. So, getting angry is a totally 'normal' response. But there's a difference between feeling angry and getting angry.

Feeling anger is a normal part of being human. Most psychologists agree that anger is a healthy emotion. Great novels have been written by angry authors in the throes of high emotion.

Mental Wellbeing and Positive Psychology for Veterinary Professionals: A Pre-emptive, Proactive and Solution-based Approach, First Edition. Laura Woodward.
© 2024 John Wiley & Sons Ltd. Published 2024 by John Wiley & Sons Ltd.

However, 'getting angry' when we become carried away with the emotion can eat us up from the inside. It can cause insomnia, unresolved stress and cardiac disease.

> *Getting angry with another person is like throwing hot coals with both hands; both people get burned.*
>
> Buddha

Showing anger in unhealthy ways can be the outward demonstration of undigested emotions by someone who lacks self-awareness and self-regulation. Not caring that we have angry outbursts directed at others shows a lack of basic good manners and a profound degree of selfishness.

Anger essentially tells our brain there is a need for quick action, short-circuiting our neural pathways, prompting a quick and often suboptimal processing of information, instead of comprehensive, systematic processing.

This processing is what we call self-regulation, and without it we may make rash decisions brought about by a surge of anger which we will regret once the feeling has subsided.

> *Speak when you are angry, and you will make the best speech you'll ever regret.*
>
> Laurence J. Peter

Is anger a temporary feeling or a perpetual state of mind or mental disorder? It varies from person to person. Most of us feel anger from time to time due to events. Some people feel background anger most of the time, often not in response to any particular stimulus. Some personality disorders make a person more likely to feel and express anger irrationally and more destructively than others.

What's Normal?

It is hard to differentiate between normal feelings of anger and unwarranted and disorderly anger.

Does 'normal' mean the healthiest mode of behaviour or behaviour that is simply representative of the majority? I reckon most of us would agree that happiness and pleasantries always trump anger and confrontation in terms of healthy and beneficial behaviour.

However, anger plays an essential role in the human emotional spectrum. Anger allows individuals to advocate for themselves and others and to avoid compromising their needs and goals in order to achieve what they want. It is the fuel behind many individuals' striving for success and has played a role in many great achievements in history. As stated by Bede Jarrett: 'The world needs anger. The world often continues to allow evil because it isn't angry enough'.

On the other hand, anger has a quintessential role in many horrific events and catastrophes. This push and pull of the benefits and consequences of anger makes it hard to determine what is an appropriate amount or level of anger.

In using our emotional intelligence which we discussed previously, *self-awareness* means we recognise when we are feeling angry. 'I am aware of situations which have angered me previously. I know what scenario is likely to anger me even before it happens. I recognise this feeling, it's anger.'

Self-regulation is where I have used the space between impulse and reaction to pause and make a conscious decision about how I want to react both outwardly and inwardly.

> *Between stimulus and response there is a space. In that space lies our power to choose our response. In our response lies our growth and freedom.*
>
> Hans Selye

By self-regulating, I know that my expression of anger, if any, is a well-thought-out action which I will take full ownership of, which will achieve what I want it to achieve and which I will not regret. It's a personal choice.

Here are some pointers to guide you.

Anger May Be Appropriate, But Rage is Not

Rage is the external symptom of unregulated anger. We've all felt the light-headed, seeing-red, violent torrent of emotion rising within. Some of us have been at the receiving end of it all too often.

While anger can be constructed into coherent arguments to reach or achieve goals, rage is destructive to the self and often to others, and without clear goals or solutions, it rarely ever achieves the solutions necessary to ease this intense emotion or dissolve the problems.

Knowing How and When to Express Your Anger is a Skill Worth Developing

Pick your battles carefully and remember that how you fight your battles makes a huge difference. For example, raising your voice will only worsen the situation because people will focus on the fact that you are yelling, not what you're yelling about.

So, if you really feel the need to say something, be sure to express yourself in a way that will allow the other person to hear you. Use good cognitive empathy to channel the energy of anger into a ferocious eloquence which cannot be ignored.

Sleep on It

Laurence J. Peter once said, 'Speak when you are angry, and you will make the best speech you'll ever regret'. As mentioned earlier, anger short-circuits the neural pathways used in thinking, so everything automatically gets simplified in your mind, becomes either black or white and as everyone knows, the world is hardly ever black or white.

> *If the only tool you have is a hammer, everything looks like a nail.*
> Abraham Maslow

The best thing to do, however difficult it may be, might be to wait it out, let your anger fall by the wayside of rationality. If you're still upset after your anger subsides, then think of a logical way to advocate for a solution to the problem. Not only will you be more confident of your right to fight, but those you are fighting against are much more likely to listen to you if you're able to argue coherently.

Anger has been the catalyst for many great and many greatly destructive events throughout the course of history. While suppressing anger can lead to resentment and embitterment, expressing it can be socially isolating, embarrassing and perhaps even socially and physically destructive.

Anger essentially forces the mind to rely on shortcuts to make rash decisions, so realising this and resisting the urge to act reactively is the first step.

Finding the place between embittered suppression and shameful destruction is the next step. A step we cannot afford to ignore.

Grief

- How to grieve mindfully
- Competitive grief
- Comparative grief

When Elisabeth Kübler-Ross wrote about what we now call the five stages of grief, denial, anger, bargaining, depression and acceptance (aka DABDA), it was her aim to describe the emotional journey of the dying person, not the bereaved.

But as the bereaved, we are desperate for something to cling on to. Something to normalise this unbearable desolation inside. Because, although we describe it as unbearable, we can't dismiss it and we have to bear it.

The loneliness of realising that grief is a personal thing and that sharing our feelings with others doesn't actually make us feel okay drives us to reach out for an explanation of how on earth it can feel so bad. So, we find an acronym for the five emotions (DABDA) and then the pain goes away?

Grief is what happens to us when we experience the loss of something which was embedded in our whole being and psyche. So, it is agony for our mind, our heart and our whole body.

Some of us are in 'the club you never want to join', where only fellow bereaved friends understand our pain. Others have yet to experience it and join this club.

When my mother died, I remember so many friends saying that they had no idea how it felt. I was so grateful for every day I had of innocence prior to knowing how bad it felt. Because nothing can prepare you for it. I felt there was no benefit to knowing.

And I noticed gratitude in me too for every day my lovely friends had without grief ripping at their hearts.

My employer at the time allowed me three days to get over it. I pleaded for more days away from work unpaid, for many reasons, one of which was that I could not actually see. As a surgeon, I was going to mess up. The firm answer was no. The practice was under unsustainable pressure because I, the surgeon, was off.

Mental Wellbeing and Positive Psychology for Veterinary Professionals: A Pre-emptive, Proactive and Solution-based Approach, First Edition. Laura Woodward.

The person telling me this had both parents still alive. I even managed to feel grateful that he had a while more before he could understand. But I'm only human. I never forgot it.

And now, six years later, my wonderful father, my confidante, my partner in bad Irish jokes is about to die. His morphine starts today. It's just a matter of days before he's gone.

Do I look away? Or can I be grateful now that I'm already in the club so I can allow these familiar feelings to be within me rather than consume me?

I'm no longer shocked at how much agony the human brain can tolerate. Wouldn't it be true self-compassion to allow myself to feel what might just break me now, rather than block those emotions out and thus seal my fate of definitely being broken by them later?

How to Grieve Mindfully

1) *Accept your feelings*: allow yourself to feel what you feel at any given moment, with a sense of self-compassion and without judgement. It's okay to be overwhelmed.

2) *Express your feelings*: just as important as accepting your feelings is expressing them. Talking won't make those feelings go away but it helps to straighten them out in your head so that they can form an orderly queue and thus be noticed one by one, defusing their hold over you with time. Wailing, sobbing, crying like you've never cried before are all 'normal' and healthy outward expressions of grief.

3) *Reach out*: during this time, it is important to reach out in multiple ways. Reach out for guidance from a counsellor or a mindfulness group. Reach out to family and distant relatives to share stories of your loved one. Reach out to offer support to other grievers. Find a balance between sitting with yourself and being with others, but ultimately, reach out – don't isolate.

4) *Continue to take care of yourself and others*: living life while grieving is another chore. It's counterintuitive to look after my body when my dad's body is failing before my eyes. It feels disrespectful and even selfish.

5) *Celebrate your loved one's life*: when my mum died, I made a thousand cups of tea like a zombie urn, as person after person came to the house to talk about mum and how wonderful she was. I remember wishing at the time that she could hear all these stories.

6) *Gratitude*: now, in my dad's final days, I am so incredibly lucky that person after person is coming to the house to talk about his life and share stories, but this time it's with him. He can chat and laugh and reminisce and, as he puts it, enjoy hearing his own eulogies before he says goodbye.

Competitive Grief

> Rather than my thinking that I have the 'one-upmanship' on bereavement, and scoff at their mildest of grief, surely I am the person best placed to understand and comfort them.

Recently, I have heard many different people talk about their emotional experiences following the death of Queen Elizabeth II. It fascinates me how many varied responses I heard, interestingly many of them deeply judgemental of others' emotional responses. But is this really a time for judgement? Or is it a time to come together in grief (be it mild or great) and to grab the opportunity to unite?

Judgement of Others

The sudden announcement of an extra bank holiday brought whoops of joy from my kids. My thoughts immediately went to my poor practice manager and the logistical nightmare this would be for her and for so many other employers and self-employed workers.

It had been planned a decade ago by Her Majesty with her understanding and acknowledgement that 25 million of her people loved her so much that they had a need (not just a desire) to watch her funeral and that, prior to that, over 250000 would want to file past her coffin as she lay in state.

The reactions from some people were of relief that they could pay their last respects to someone with whom they felt a deep connection. One of my colleagues said she would cry if she couldn't watch the funeral. Another said that she would cry if she saw any snippet of the funeral anywhere. Such were some of the varied reactions to the death of the Queen.

What struck me most is that, for some people, this is the greatest grief they have ever felt. And just because others of us have seen our parents die, which is such horrible, life-changing, heart-shredding grief, that doesn't negate the fact that this may be the greatest grief the other person has ever felt.

Who are we to say 'You think that's bad? You should feel this'?
Grief is not a competition.

The person who cried hysterically when the Queen died did not make my grief worse. It was already as bad as it gets. So why should I deny them their need for comfort and understanding? How would their stiff upper lip have made my parents any less dead? It wouldn't.

So, if someone wails at the news that the Queen has died, stays in bed crying for days, queues for more days to see her coffin and then spends a day watching her laid to rest, rather than my thinking that I have the 'one-upmanship' on bereavement, and scoff at their mildest of grief, surely I am the person best placed to understand them.

Similarly, if I am the oracle on grief because I've 'been there twice', then I should have understanding in abundance of their feelings and be able to comfort them easily.

Comparative Grief

Six years ago, when my mother died, I was distraught. She was 80 and amazing. It still strikes me as funny that, as soon as people know your mum has died, they rapidly follow with the question 'How old was she?'. To those of us in 'the club you never want to join' aka the dead parents club, her age was of no significance on a scale of things at the time. Now I understand that it is the questioner's reflexive and clumsy attempt to make it 'okay'. 'They lived a good life' or my least favourite 'At least they had a good innings'. My parents had less than no interest in cricket.

What I remember more clearly from that time, surprisingly with warmth and with comfort, was how there were three of us 'recently bereaved' parents at the school gates every afternoon at pick-up time. The other woman's sister had died of cancer at the age of 40. The man's son had died of a brain tumour at 19.

And yet, while my mum's death was the natural order of older people dying before younger ones, neither the other woman nor the man belittled my grief as less than theirs. I was humbled to receive their hugs and comfort even though I felt that their grief was more tragic and 'wrong' compared to mine. They, however, felt that grief is so unbelievably awful, there is literally no way to measure it. So, we were all equal.

Just as the expanse of the infinite universe is immeasurable and beyond human comprehension, so too, sometimes, is the infinite pain we feel when our loved ones die.

Grief brought us together in this club.

Rather than judging others for weeping upon the death of the Queen, we could use this time as an opportunity to bond rather than judge others for their depth of emotion.

The Queue

What a spectacle. What a symbol of true, idiosyncratic Britishness. I wondered if the satellites shifted their view of the Great Wall of China and instead focused on this massive gathering of stoically patient people united in grief despite their differences.

Friends were made in The Queue, even romances started in it. There was sharing of stories, food and blankets in The Queue.

Her Majesty brought people of every culture together in that perfectly snaking line. It had been orchestrated by Professor Keith Still, a crowd science expert, and his team of Crowd Science Masters students with the authorisation of Queen Elizabeth.

There was even a queue to join the queue to join The Queue. All planned a decade in advance.

Some people queued for over 24 hours to see the Queen lie in state. Some flew across the Atlantic to join The Queue. I saw that one man queued twice to see her lie in state, and he was overjoyed he managed to do this. Each time he walked through Westminster Hall he had a different experience, he said.

People said it was the best day of their life, the greatest thing they ever did. Others said it brought them closure from complicated long-term grief for a loved one. Others felt it was a pilgrimage of sorts on behalf of a dead loved one. I couldn't see any report of anyone regretting it or having a 'meh' moment afterwards.

A few days later, I listened to someone who said it had made their 'blood boil' to see people cry hysterically when Princess Diana died. Few other scenarios come to mind where our blood boils with anger because someone is crying and distraught. It has to be this competitive grief which causes the anger and judgement.

And yet, feeling this blood-boiling anger and disdain for others will never bring us peace.

I'm just suggesting that we look inside ourselves and find a place where we can forgive others for feeling grief which is less painful than our own.

The Emotional Burden of Error

- Guilt
- Fear
- Isolation

> When things go wrong, the experiences of the pet owners and those of the vets may be strikingly similar and yet damagingly divisive.

Involvement in errors often results in serious health effects and emotional distress, as well as performance and work-related consequences for staff members and in particular the vet in charge of the case.

We've all been there: the sickening feeling in the pit of your stomach when you see that you have failed. The guilt and shame can be all-consuming. Fear of our inability to manage the case can prevent us from being able to help this patient at all. And the loneliness of knowing this is all your fault is very isolating.

Sometimes, our distress prevents us from reaching out to the very people who are feeling similar emotions at that time – the owners.

Guilt

Though it is well recognised that vets feel guilty after making mistakes, owners often have similar or even stronger feelings of guilt.

Despite acknowledging that they probably could not have prevented the error, owners often berate themselves and feel guilty about not keeping close enough watch. 'Maybe I should have gone to another vet', 'Maybe I shouldn't have consented to the surgery', 'My dog trusted me, and I let her down.'

Although full disclosure of errors is increasingly recognised as an ethical imperative, vets often shy away from taking personal responsibility for an error and believe they must 'choose words carefully' or present a positive 'spin'. Most practices do not perform revision surgery free of charge because it's an 'admission of guilt'. However, maybe a healthier approach is to admit to the fault and still charge for the revision surgery.

Mental Wellbeing and Positive Psychology for Veterinary Professionals: A Pre-emptive, Proactive and Solution-based Approach, First Edition. Laura Woodward.
© 2024 John Wiley & Sons Ltd. Published 2024 by John Wiley & Sons Ltd.

Otherwise the result can be an impersonal demeanour that leads patients to view the practice as uncaring.

Charging makes economic sense and the clients should have been advised in advance that complications are a real possibility and that the treatment of such will be chargeable.

The last thing we need when feeling guilty is the added stress of hiding the guilt from the client and then running the risk of them turning to Doctor Google and the inevitable backlash that can cause.

In the medical profession, approximately 30 US states have adopted 'I'm sorry' laws, which to varying degrees render comments that doctors make to patients after an error inadmissible as evidence for proving liability.

Until such statutes become universal, frightened clinicians are left to struggle with conflicting personal moral principles, professional ethics and institutional policies.

Fear

Often the pet owner fears that if they question the expertise or skill of the vet, especially after an error, because of the power dynamics between vets and pet owners, their pet may experience further harm or neglect. Fear of retribution or of future poor treatment because of asking questions about mistakes must be unbearable for a pet owner at a time when they are at their most vulnerable. And yet we, consumed by our own guilt and fear, may be too self-obsessed to empathise with this client.

Vets who feel guilty after a medical error may have parallel feelings of fear – fear for their reputation, their job and their own future as well as that of their patient.

Isolation

Given the nature of the emotions provoked by the error, feelings of isolation can be particularly harmful. Pet owners say that at times like this, they need someone involved in the case to reach out to them and connect with them, no matter how painful.

The vet at the same time is suffering alone, agonising over the harm they have caused, the loss of their pet owner's trust, the loss of their colleagues' respect, their diminished self-confidence and the potential effects of the error on their career.

When vets and nurses back away from patients and their owners, it may be because of their own feelings of guilt, fear and isolation, compounded by legal or institutional advice. Paralysed by shame or lacking in their own understanding of why the error occurred, vets may find a truthful conversation too awkward. They may also be unwilling or unable to talk to anyone about the event, inhibiting both their learning and the likelihood of achieving resolution. Such avoidance and silence compound the harm. What many owners want is *more* communication, not less. They will still experience guilt, fear and sadness but by putting our feelings aside for a moment, at least we can make them feel less alone.

So how can we accept that complications can and do occur (which we want our clients to accept) and be able to remain professional, caring and mentally strong when it happens? Surely honest and direct communication is the most important antidote to guilt, fear and isolation. Silence and evasion breed distrust. Pet owners don't want spin doctors either at a time like this.

They certainly do not want a cover-up. They want compassion, they want to understand their situation fully and to know what the event has taught the practice. They want as much communication as you can possibly give, however painful it may be for you to phone them twice a week for months on end.

When things go wrong, the experiences of pet owners and those of vets may be strikingly similar and yet damagingly divisive. Although apology and disclosure are necessary, they may be insufficient to elicit forgiveness, which encompasses shared understanding, rekindled trust, acceptance and closure. Everyone involved needs an organised structure that restores communication and supports emotional needs.

So what would such a structure look like?

- Morbidity and mortality rounds on a monthly basis help to remove the stigma from making errors and are paramount if we are to prevent further similar errors.
- 'First responders' in a practice, who are usually staff members with a cursory training in mental health first aid, should be deployed when an error occurs to guide the vets, nurses and pet owners through the

plethora of ensuing emotions and keep communication open, honest and plentiful.

- Regular mental wellbeing seminars for the whole practice to help build emotional intelligence and resilience in professions which have to accept that to err is human.
- One-to-one counselling for individuals who are struggling to cope or even just 'not thriving'.

Success is not a good teacher. Failure makes you humble.
Shah Rukh Khan

Guilt

- I feel guilty
- What is guilt?
- Misuse of guilt
- Helpful guilt
- Misplaced guilt

Sometimes it's difficult to be upbeat when we're aware of the suffering of others even though they may be unknown to us. For example, during the COVID-19 pandemic, people all over the planet were suffering. And yet, some of us weren't. It was easy to feel guilty for feeling okay during that time. Or during the war in Ukraine, other global crises, famine, floods, tsunamis in other countries far away from ours, again, anonymous people's lives are being destroyed and ours are continuing quite mundanely with commuting to work, grocery shopping and planning our weekends.

Closer to home, many of us are pet owners as well as veterinary professionals. We understand the anxiety, worry and sadness of our clients and often it is us who have made them anxious, worried and sad.

When we have our vet or vet nurse hat on, explaining to our clients what needs to be done next, giving them estimates which will be more than they can afford or delivering other bad news can make us feel guilty. Maybe it's because *we* don't have to feel the pain we've inflicted on them or maybe because we are going home to our healthy pet.

I experienced this recently when I brought my ageing, skinny and polydipsic cat into work for the team to diagnose and treat. I had procrastinated for so long, possibly because I didn't want to know the truth about my beloved cat. I entrusted her to the kind arms of my two closest nurses and my gentle, knowledgeable, medical colleague vet.

I could feel the conflicting emotions in that vet as he delivered the blood and urine results to me over the phone: kindness, sadness for me and overwhelming guilt for making me distraught.

Then I felt guilt along with my grief; guilt because I had put my wonderful colleagues in that position of processing the samples and delivering horrible news to me.

Mental Wellbeing and Positive Psychology for Veterinary Professionals: A Pre-emptive, Proactive and Solution-based Approach, First Edition. Laura Woodward.
© 2024 John Wiley & Sons Ltd. Published 2024 by John Wiley & Sons Ltd.

Then they all went home and felt guilty because their cats were just fine compared to mine, and I took my cat home and felt guilty because I'd put her through a day in the hospital.

The contradictions in our minds between enjoying and even loving our life and knowing all the while that people worldwide and down the road and in our practice are suffering can bring on guilt. Other times, guilt might be just one of the many uncomfortable unidentified emotions grumbling along in the background of our minds.

I Feel Guilty

Being self-aware is the first competency of emotional intelligence, so recognising that you are feeling guilty is helpful and a good place to start. Now, what to do with these feelings? As self-awareness is the first, then self-regulation is the second, i.e. our reactions to this emotion are totally within our control.

What is Guilt?

Guilt is a wired-in emotion evoked when we believe we have done something bad or when we feel undeserving of our good fortune. It's quite a complex emotion, and an inhibitory one. For example, if I have done something unkind to another person, I may feel guilty afterwards. This overriding emotion can block out the other additional emotions which could otherwise arise, such as anger towards that person, anger towards myself, or selfishness and lack of caring about others.

The evolutionary purpose of guilt is to keep us positively connected to others. It's an advantage for humans to work together, so it's important that we have an emotion to override selfishness. Guilt pushes us to stay in the good graces of the people we need. The uncomfortable physical feeling that guilt evokes propels us to do the less harmful thing next time or to make amends.

That was good for when we were living in small tribes and engaging with our neighbours all day every day in the hunter-gatherer phase of evolution. Back then, it was of paramount importance to remain in the good graces of our fellow tribe members or we would be ostracised and starve.

These days, when we are unlikely to be living in a tribe, and if we have enough self-regulation that we can inhibit our own angry outbursts and selfishness, guilt may be one emotion worthy of being examined, faced and then let go of.

On the other hand, maybe you have indeed done something unkind to another, and the guilt is serving its purpose of making you question your behaviour and change it.

Misuse of Guilt

Guilt can be 'misused'. For example, if I express out loud to others that I am feeling guilty or ashamed about the way I acted, then that can be an attempt to absolve myself of all responsibility for what I have done rather than face the uncomfortable facts that I have transgressed and need to take action.

Grand confessions are a misuse of guilt and achieve little in the way of self-improvement.

Narcissists typically use elaborate grand confessions to express their pseudo guilt to others, to evoke sympathy from the masses, rather than welcoming their friends' constructive criticism which could be painful. The subsequent reassurance and congratulations for their humility (albeit fake) provide the much needed validation the narcissist craves in order to cope with the world.

Helpful Guilt

Helpful guilt can be useful when it's the driving force to make amends for something truly bad that we have done to another. Once our emotionally intelligent self has identified that what we are feeling is guilt, it can be the impetus for change to becoming a better person. Self-flagellation and self-deprecation will achieve less than examining our feelings of shame closely and identifying how to become a better person as a result.

Misplaced Guilt

Guilt can be 'misplaced'. For example, the misplaced guilt we feel for having limits when it comes to helping others is very different from the useful guilt we may have after knowingly being unkind to another person.

Helping others is noble. Doing it to such a degree that you are exhausted mentally and physically is unwise and can lead to burnout.

Identifying your feeling of misplaced guilt is the place to start if you are to use it in a positive way.

Self-preservation is of paramount importance if you are to keep yourself healthy while being a helpful member of your family and of society. Everyone has limits to how much they can give of themselves before it starts to become a drain on their resources. Being mindful and noticing this limit is essential for good mental wellbeing.

The metaphor of putting your own oxygen mask on before helping others with theirs may be overused, but it's still relevant. I cannot help others if I am running on empty.

Acceptance of your uncomfortable yet self-preserving guilty feelings will paradoxically help you to feel less 'bad'.

Transforming Misplaced Guilt into Something Beneficial

One way is to shift from guilt to gratitude – here's how you do it.

Think about what you have done that makes you feel guilty. If you know that guilt is misplaced, focus on trying to feel grateful for it.

For example, 'I feel guilty for making that client cry when I told her that her cat has renal failure'.

I experience my guilt as a sinking feeling in my stomach reaching down to my toes.

Now I shift into gratitude, e.g. 'I'm grateful I can give her a diagnosis, which was her aim in bringing her cat to me'.

Without being saccharine or joining the 'turn that frown upside down' brigade, if you identify your guilt as misplaced, there will always be a way to transform it. But it does take effort.

Another example: 'That client's dog will never be truly comfortable on that leg after an open articular fracture. But my own dog is 100% sound'.

Provided the treatment was good and evidence based, sometimes the trauma results in a degree of arthritis.

Examine the guilt. Once you establish that the procedure was of good quality, and that the residual mild lameness is indeed because the joint was openly scraped along the tarmac and full of bitumen when you saw it, you can put this in the misplaced guilt category and then choose to let it go and shift to gratitude.

For example, 'I'm grateful that was her only injury, that I saw her swiftly and that I have a large knowledge base at my fingertips and the correct equipment to do a good fracture repair'.

Also, 'I'm grateful it wasn't my dog who had that horrific injury'.

Shifting misplaced guilt is not about saying 'Never mind, at least .....' at every hurdle. It is specifically for when we have identified our feelings as guilt, and then as misplaced guilt.

Gratitude is so much more useful to us and to others than misplaced guilt. However, helpful guilt can be our moral compass. Identifying which type of guilt we are feeling is the place to start.

When Your World Falls Apart

What if you're in the place where your worst fears become a reality? When life suddenly becomes unbearable.

For example, when your parent has been ill for a long time and their hospital visits and medications have become the norm. All that time, you are in a heightened state of anxiety without even realising it because it's normal. This might go on for years.

Then the worst happens. The very worst. They actually die. You never knew that that could actually happen. Your world falls apart as theirs ends.

What if your relationship has been a bit off for so long that you accept it as the normal stage of your relationship right now? Many together-forever couples do move from crazy head-spinning times to settled comfortable times, to years when they're happiest spending small amounts of time together.

It might be that you've been in an increased state of anxiety or stress for years even though you're still together. All this time, you're hypercoagulable and hypertensive, rarely taking a full conscious breath. Then the relationship ends and it's like you've been on a cliff edge for so long you can't remember being anywhere else. And then the sky comes crashing down on you and sends you falling into the chasm over the cliff.

When you're going through hell, for goodness sake keep going.

What if you've been trying to have a child for so long that your life consists of calendars and 28-day cycles and little else? Then you get pregnant and then you miscarry.

It's sheer and utter hell. You find it impossible to believe anyone has ever survived such horrors.

How on earth can soft mindfulness bring any comfort or coping abilities when your life is in such turmoil?

In the *Canadian Journal of Psychiatry*, a study by Farb et al. (2012) explains how people who meditate are more able to tolerate their own distress than people who don't. One part of the prefrontal cortex associated with stress regulation is the anterior cingulate cortex (ACC). Poor ACC function tends to correlate with impulsive behaviour and mental inflexibility – which are both common among people under stress.

Mental Wellbeing and Positive Psychology for Veterinary Professionals: A Pre-emptive, Proactive and Solution-based Approach, First Edition. Laura Woodward.

Experienced meditators display more activity in the ACC and better stress regulation (Taren et al. 2015).

As veterinary professionals, we're good at creating problem lists, triaging them and problem solving, or at least problem management.

We use flow diagrams, spider diagrams and spreadsheets to calm our minds at work. We have checklists to force our minds to stay focused and clear in a crisis. We can also use these tools when the crisis is our life.

Mindfulness encourages us to focus on the present moment as if our life depended on it. And yet the present moment is so painful, I just want to be unconscious, drunk or asleep.

But this agony isn't going anywhere soon. Sleep helps to pass the time and allows us to feel a bit more rested. Eating and drinking water are important to function and we need to function.

Then taking time to form problem lists and spreadsheets is so helpful, and second nature to us, that at least giving it a go isn't going to make things worse. Things are already as bad as we believe they can be.

When someone dies, whatever their religious affiliation or without any affiliation, there are a known series of steps which have to happen. Hospital and hospice staff, undertakers, powers of attorney, executors of wills and others just appear out of nowhere and walk us through those steps.

I'll be forever grateful to the people in the funeral home for literally walking me and my children through the steps of what we needed to do, where we needed to be at what time and which car to sit in. They provided water, umbrellas, kindness, silence and a pen and paper for our eulogies. They held our hands.

When our relationship or our dream job ends, there are no undertakers and funeral home staff to hold our hands. It may be that the person who used to hold our hand and helped us to navigate these nightmares is gone with the relationship or the workplace. It's even lonelier than bereavement sometimes. And yet it feels like a bereavement, and we have to grieve.

How do I combine problem solving with mindfulness? There are many ways. No way is more correct than the other. The more you make it your own plan, the more valid and empowering it is.

At this time, when you have no power or energy, anything which restarts your power bank is probably helpful.

Because we are often literally clueless when our world falls apart, I'm going to suggest one way of combining mindfulness and problem solving like the hearse driver did for me; laying it out one step at a time, clear as day, so I didn't fall over.

With an A4 notebook, you could make several problem lists and triage them.

1) For example, one page could be about urgent problems for today, e.g. how do I get from A to B?

    How do I prepare for work or do I call in absent?

    I need food and water.

    I need sleep.

    Things I don't need, e.g. social media, news apps, melancholy break-up songs.

    List these problems in a column on one side of the page and ideally make this page a few pages into the book rather than the first page. I'll explain why later.

2) The next page can be a list of problems for tomorrow, for example clothes, food and water, people I have to contact urgently.

    Again, list these on one side.

3) The next page can be problems/targets for the next week, for example arrangements in case of bereavement. Notifying landlords if I have to move out. Organising my CV if my job ends.

4) Another page can be a list of worries about the future.

    How will I ever love or trust someone again?

    I'm never going to have a child.

    How will I ever find a secure job again?

    What if I've made a terrible mistake?

    How will I afford the bills?

    These problems will loom large. You can allow yourself to 'awfulise' here. We've talked about the dangers associated with awfulising before but it would be naïve to think that a life crisis won't give rise to awfulising, so let's not judge ourselves for it just now.

5) Next, on this page, make a column in the middle of the page and list the emotions and physical feelings each problem causes.

    Next to 'how will I ever love or trust someone again?', you might write the emotions of loneliness, desolation, terror or the physical feelings of chest ache, sleepwalking, disassociation.

Please write down what you feel. Take some time to close your eyes, breathe and examine the feelings you have about each individual thing. Make a long list. Try to give each feeling at least 10 breaths.

6) Then, on the far side of the page, you can write any strategies or ideas you may have for dealing with each problem, apart from noticing it and the feelings it causes. This list will be added to, and crossed out as time passes. You might leave it blank.

There are probably no strategies for 'fixing' the terror of feeling unlovable but there are ideas you will have about paying the bills. Now we're going to work our way backwards through the notebook.

7) Going back to the previous page of problems/targets for the next week, this is often a much easier page to work through when it comes to strategies.

Your practical mind might come to play here, which can feel empowering. If you have any inkling of empowerment and if you notice that your mind is calming down by untangling this plethora of problems and feelings, try to stop, take a breath and make that feeling as prominent and long lasting as you can.

Notifying the landlord that you're moving out and designing headstones for the grave make it very real and final, and that can be indescribably painful. The more time you spend acknowledging that pain, the faster it will dissipate. Crying is a normal human reaction to intense pain. Allowing yourself this physical reaction to the emotions you're naming is part of your grieving, your self-care and your recovery.

8) The pages of problems for tomorrow and today are emergency care. This is often about getting through it because you have no other option.

You never know how strong you are until being strong is the only choice you have.

Bob Marley

You might have no emotions about organising food, water and travel for today and tomorrow. You may feel numb and in shock and like an android. Write these down if you can. Physically, you might feel nauseous, exhausted, hungry, not hungry. Again, the more you put feelings into words and acknowledge them by writing them down, the easier they are to bear.

When my children were small, if they had problems and wanted to chat, they would tend to blurt out everything in what seemed like one breath. A brain dump. Then they would look to me for answers.

As a child and adolescent counsellor, I knew that giving them all the solutions (my solutions) would do more to disempower them than to help them. So, I devised a way to help them.

As they spoke, I would listen actively and intently, then I would write it down. It was this act of writing it down that made them feel recognised and validated.

Then, we'd have a long pause, sometimes bewilderingly long. Then pretty much every time, they would then produce a solution, their solution, whether it was a practical thing they would do or an acceptance of it – it varied all the time. Their eyes were fresh and their minds uncluttered. I learnt from them and their insight more than they learnt from me in those times.

In a way, mindfulness encourages us to see things with wonder and fresh eyes, like a child. Children are naturally mindful and caught up in the present moment for most of their early years. That's why many of them have an easier life compared to us adults.

Adopting that awe and curiosity at a time of crisis can help with these flow diagrams and spreadsheets.

Writing them down is a bit like journalling for vets and nurses with our own spin on it and using our own inherent talents.

Over the next few weeks, you can add to all of these pages and subtract from them as well. Your way of thinking and your ideas may evolve rapidly.

9) When you feel like it, you can add in a page or more at the beginning of your book which you kept blank at the start. This can be about your regrets or mourning or question marks about the past. For example, you might feel like those years in your relationship or all those attempts at IVF have been wasted.

You might have regrets about not spending more time with your loved one who's dead. That's how you feel now. There will be lists of emotions and physical feelings on this page. There probably aren't any solutions to these things from the past and that's partly why I feel it's something to examine when the immediate crisis has passed but it's your choice.

This isn't going to help everyone. But it definitely does help some people.

References

Farb, N.A., Anderson, A.K., and Segal, Z.V. (2012). The mindful brain and emotion regulation in mood disorders. *Canadian Journal of Psychiatry* 57 (2): 70–77.

Taren, A.A., Gianaros, P.J., Greco, C.M. et al. (2015). Mindfulness meditation training alters stress-related amygdala resting state functional connectivity: a randomized controlled trial. *Social Cognitive and Affective Neuroscience* 10 (12): 1758–1768.

Euthanasia and Suicide

Whether we view our ability to euthanase our patients as a privilege or as a horrific part of our job, at one stage or another we will be actively involved in ending the lives of some of our patients.

Is this a precursor to depression and other mental health difficulties we have as veterinary professionals? Or is it even a precursor to our own suicide?

We will all have different opinions, but evidence-based study conclusions are there to answer at least some of our queries.

We have evidence that vets are more likely to experience mood disorders and suicide than other occupational groups (Fritschi et al. 2009). The studies in this reference are from over a decade ago but few studies of this kind have been published, so I'm referring to them for evidence.

Being dated, I note that many if the reports did not include vet nurses. However, we need to assume that if these studies were conducted today, the results would reflect all veterinary professionals and not just the vets.

As an aside, what is striking is that our shocking mental health records have been known and proven for several decades. Therefore, it's safe to assume that we're not doing enough, or enough of the right things, to effect change.

> However much of our budget is allocated to tackling the mental health crises of our staff, we're not doing enough or enough of the right things to effect change. If we were, our suicide rate would be decreasing.

Performing euthanasia of our patients has been implicated as contributing to the prevalence of suicide risk and psychological distress in veterinarians (Bartram and Baldwin 2008). However, more thorough studies show that while performing euthanasia does indeed contribute to some of our mental health problems, it can actually decrease our risk of suicide.

Fogle and Abrahamson (1990) examined the possible negative impact that performing euthanasia may have on vets. They and others proposed that performing euthanasia could potentially influence our development of depression, suicidal ideation and suicidal behaviours. They suggest that the performance of euthanasia may promote more favourable attitudes towards human euthanasia, end of life and the expendability of life.

Jones-Fairnie et al. (2008) found that suicidal *ideation* (where we consider suicide as a solution to our problems) is more related to other factors such as depression than it is to our ease of access to means. However, we know that access to means is likely to be why our suicide *rate* is twice that of doctors and dentists (Petersen and Burnett 2008).

Hawton and van Heeringen (2009) proposed that this access to lethal medications is the reason why we move so quickly from suicidal ideation to actual suicidal behaviour.

Performing euthanasia is desperately upsetting for us as the carers of our patients. We grieve for those pets and feel a huge sense of loss when they are gone. We empathise with their owners who are in psychological distress. We give of ourselves to them before and after, having long and painful conversations often with many family members before the event and answering calls long after the euthanasia, because they need reassurance that they did the right thing. It's truly horrible. Of course, this is affecting us.

But surprisingly, Bartram and Baldwin (2010) show that overall euthanasia *frequency* plays a minimal role in our rates of depression (1% of the total variation when other factors, such as age, etc., are taken into consideration). It's other factors which determine how depressed we are.

Also, performing euthanasia is not something which increases our rates of suicide. In fact, ironically, one study shows that it *decreases* the likelihood of us moving from depression to suicide (Tran et al. 2014). Why is this? Perhaps it is because of our clients showing us their raw grief and pain that we suddenly realise the impact our death would have on those left behind. That is, we move from the egocentricism that often accompanies depression to taking a step back to observe as an onlooker and see that there are more people to consider apart from just us.

It may be because, when we are suffering from depression, we sometimes don't truly appreciate the finality and irreversibility of death until we see it in front of us (Allberg and Chu 1990).

So, while access to euthanasia drugs is a significant factor in our high suicide rate, it's not necessarily performing euthanasia which brought us to that hopeless place. Knowing that performing euthanasia is only slightly affecting vets' mental wellbeing, it isn't increasing their suicide risk and it may even be acting as a buffer between those with suicidal ideation and actual suicide may bring us some comfort.

But discussion around our very long-term and unresolving mental health difficulties isn't designed to bring us comfort. It's designed to wake us up to this dire situation which isn't getting any better. With this in mind, I would like to bring to our attention the converse.

If performing euthanasia acts as a buffer between us and our own suicide, it would be wise to observe the potentially increased risk of suicide amongst those of us *not* used to performing euthanasia with any frequency, e.g. surgeons, specialists and nurses.

Proactively tackling that risk could bring some comfort.

References

Allberg, W.R. and Chu, L. (1990). Understanding adolescent suicide: correlates in a developmental perspective. *School Counsellor* 37: 343–351.

Bartram, D.J. and Baldwin, D.S. (2008). Veterinary surgeons and suicide: influences, opportunities and research directions. *Veterinary Record* 162: 36–40.

Bartram, D.J. and Baldwin, D.S. (2010). Veterinary surgeons and suicide: a structured review of the possible influences on increased risk. *Veterinary Record* 166: 388–397.

Fogle, B. and Abrahamson, D. (1990). Pet loss: a survey of the attitudes and feelings of practicing veterinarians. *Anthrozoös* 3: 143–150.

Fritschi, L., Morrison, D., Shirangi, A., and Day, L. (2009). Psychological wellbeing of Australian veterinarians. *Australian Veterinary Journal* 87: 76–81.

Hawton, K. and van Heeringen, K. (2009). Suicide. *Lancet* 373: 1372–1381.

Jones-Fairnie, H., Ferroni, P., Silburn, S., and Lawrence, D. (2008). Suicide in Australian veterinarians. *Australian Veterinary Journal* 86: 114–116.

Petersen, M.R. and Burnett, C.A. (2008). The suicide mortality of working physicians and dentists. *Occupational Medicine* 58: 25–29.

Tran, L., Crane, M.F., and Phillips, J.K. (2014). The distinct role of performing euthanasia on depression and suicide in veterinarians. *Journal of Occupational Health Psychology* 19 (2): 123–132.

Chronic Pain

Many of us will experience chronic pain at some point in our lives. The definition of 'chronic' varies for each of us, perhaps as a reflection of the psychological impact the pain has on us as individuals. For some people, chronic pain may mean a headache that lasted for a week. For others, chronic pain may mean the relentless central nervous system wind-up as a result of permanent rheumatoid arthritis in multiple joints. It's not a competition, though.

The effect of mindfulness in the management of chronic pain has been debated for decades. It is difficult to measure people's degree of mindfulness, especially when not in a meditative state.

What we can measure, using a fMRI scan, is the activity in the different areas of the brain responsible for cognition, emotion, reasoning, etc. and how they respond to a known painful stimulus.

- *The brains of meditators respond differently to pain.* Grant and Rainville (2009) used functional and structural MRI to ascertain the brain mechanisms involved in mindfulness-related pain reduction. They found that during pain, meditators (albeit in a non-meditative state while being studied) had *increased* activation in areas associated with processing the actual sensory experience of pain (including primary and secondary somatosensory areas, insula, thalamus and midcingulate cortex). They also found *decreased* activity in regions involved in emotion, memory and appraisal (including medial prefrontal cortex, orbital frontal cortex, amygdala, caudate and hippocampus).
- *Activation of different neural pathways from placebo.* Zeidan et al. (2015) found mostly consistent results and went a step further and accomplished the feat of proving that mindfulness meditation has a different neural pathway from a placebo. Also, that mindfulness reduces pain intensity above and beyond a placebo effect. In this study, relative to other comparison groups, mindfulness meditation was associated with decreased activity in the thalamus. This possibly reflects the inability of sensory information to reach areas of the brain associated with thinking and evaluation.

So should we try mindfulness or opioids? Both.

Mental Wellbeing and Positive Psychology for Veterinary Professionals: A Pre-emptive, Proactive and Solution-based Approach, First Edition. Laura Woodward.
© 2024 John Wiley & Sons Ltd. Published 2024 by John Wiley & Sons Ltd.

Mindfulness-based stress reduction (MBSR – see Part Four, Chapter 2) uses mindfulness to perceive pain from a non-judgemental perspective. It doesn't claim to reduce pain but rather to reduce the suffering experienced as a result of intractable pain.

In 1985, Jon Kabat-Zinn studied 90 chronic pain patients who were trained in MBSR. That seems far too small a group and too long ago to influence current professionals who base their decisions on real-time evidence-based studies. However, the results indicated statistically significant reductions in measures of present-moment pain, negative body image, inhibition of activity by pain, mood disturbance and psychological symptoms such as anxiety and depression. Also, opioid self-medication doses were voluntarily reduced amongst the group.

The mechanisms behind how MBSR works to reduce the suffering caused by pain aren't mysterious or magic.

Mindfulness trains us in the ability to put a space between the objective sensory elements of pain and the subjective judgement that we have of the pain.

If you have a pain, any pain, try for a moment to list all the feelings you have regarding that discomfort. Write them down. Then see if you can divide them into two lists, one list being the physical elements of the pain, e.g. shooting pains, constant ache, the other being the psychological and emotional feelings which the pain has caused, e.g. frustration, worry, anxiety, yearning for it to go away, striving to find a solution, etc.

Which list is longer?

Most people find that the psychological list has many more elements to it, which is great news really. This is because we can do something about the things on this list to reduce the impact they have on our quality of life.

Pain is a complex phenomenon due to it being a subjective and multi-dimensional experience with sensory and cognitive elements.

When we first experience pain, we usually jump to the instant judgement of it being 'bad' and something which must be extinguished. As veterinary professionals, we are masters of analgesia with an enviable array of drugs in our personal pharmacies and an enormous arsenal of other drugs in our practices. Most of our physically painful experiences are short-lived as a result.

So, when the long-term pain arrives, with its resistance to our drugs, its obstinacy, its persistence, the actual sensations are compounded by the frustrations it causes. How dare this pain escape my cures? We may be angry, yearning for it to stop, exhausted by trying to diagnose and cure it.

Ironically, the psychological pain enhances the suffering and distress caused by the original stimulus (the pain) and we try to escape it all with excessive use of alcohol, opioids, double-dose NSAIDs, anything rather than be beaten by the monster we have created out of the pain we judged.

Mindfulness meditation can be used to create more awareness of the sensation of pain itself, without judgement or resistance. This sounds counterproductive.

Jon Kabat-Zinn defines mindfulness as paying attention, on purpose, to the present moment non-judgementally. By paying attention to the site of our pain with full focus on the physical sensations and deciding that we do not have to judge them as bad, good, anything, it's a start.

Then, allowing yourself to notice the emotional sensations it gives rise to, one at a time, focusing on each emotion for as long as possible, you can distinguish between the physical sensations and the psychological sensations a bit better.

As we discussed before, often just noticing an emotion, looking it in the eyes for as long as you possibly can, giving it a name and then allowing it to pass by defuses its hold on you. Thus, we can reduce this monster. Notice that we aren't trying to stop the pain; we are merely managing our reactions to it.

When we become more aware of what we are actually experiencing, without the overlay of our judgement, the overall perception of pain is reduced.

Ironically, accepting the discomfort and being quietly aware of its presence sometimes makes the monster skulk away. Or at least seem a bit less monstrous.

References

Grant, J.A. and Rainville, P. (2009). Pain sensitivity and analgesic effects of mindful states in Zen meditators: a cross-sectional study. *Psychosomatic Medicine* 71: 106–114.

Zeidan, F., Emerson, N., Farris, S. et al. (2015). Mindfulness meditation-based pain relief employs different neural mechanisms than placebo and sham mindfulness meditation-induced analgesia. *Journal of Neuroscience* 35 (46): 15307–15325.

Burnout

- The three dimensions of burnout
- Emotional exhaustion (focus, language and posture)
- Depersonalisation
- Disconnection from purpose
- Summary of burnout

- Neuroplasticity and reversing burnout
- The evidence base
- Recognising burnout
- Suicide, burnout and chronic stress
- Mindfulness and burnout
- Mindfulness mentality and change

We're constantly hearing about burnout in the media, amongst ourselves, from colleagues, NHS workers too. But what exactly is it and how do I know if I'm burnt out? Or if I'm slowly burning out unbeknown to myself?

Even if you are suffering from burnout, and even if you can see the symptoms in yourself, do not presume that it's 'game over'. On the contrary, recognising these symptoms with self-awareness is an enlightenment and a sign that there can be a change coming and there is hope.

Deciding not to throw in the towel is self-regulation. Reading on is motivation.

Let's take a look at you in this moment, in privacy.

There are three dimensions to burnout.

The Three Dimensions of Burnout

- *Emotional exhaustion* characterised by a disconnection from joy.
- *Depersonalisation* where you feel removed from your emotions and like an onlooker into your life.
- *Disconnection from purpose* where you feel like your life is going nowhere or is even pointless.

Let's look a bit deeper into these dimensions.

Mental Wellbeing and Positive Psychology for Veterinary Professionals: A Pre-emptive, Proactive and Solution-based Approach, First Edition. Laura Woodward.
© 2024 John Wiley & Sons Ltd. Published 2024 by John Wiley & Sons Ltd.

Emotional Exhaustion (Focus, Language and Posture)

Your emotional state is made up of three things.

- Where your *focus* is. Check now where your focus is. Is it all over the place? Is it rehashing the past, organising or worrying about the future? Is it multitasking like normal but that's just a regular day? Is it focused on reading this and nothing else? Where's your phone? Just notice where your focus is non-judgementally.
- What *language* you're using in that moment. Consider the language you have been using in your internal chatter for the last few hours. Try to remember what words you have been using.
- What your *body* is doing. Observe your body: posture, comfort or discomfort, hungry, caffeine high or low? Observe your breathing rate and depth, your heart rate. Notice everything you can about your present physical sensations.

Remember your present emotional state right now is related to your focus, language and body.

> You can learn to switch your body's physiology from chaos to coherence in milliseconds.

You can adjust your emotional state to a large degree by being proactive. It's not easy, and often, if you're sad or depressed, it can be impossible. But being *aware* of the possibility is helpful even if you don't act upon it.

Focus

With focus, using the meditations on pages 58–62 and the mini-meditations on pages 67 and 68, you can gain a clearer view of what you need to focus on and what you want to focus on at this moment. You can use the imagery on pages 69 and 70 to 'open the shutters'. You can then decide what is in your view for this moment.

It takes practice. The more you train your mind to focus, the less tangled your thoughts become. It's learning to take charge of where your focus is in order to have some control over your emotional state.

> You are not a prisoner of your mind. You can be in partnership with it.

A good method I use with my clients to train your mind to start the day untangled is to 'be in the shower when you're in the shower'. In that inspirational as well as humorous interview with Oprah, Jon Kabat-Zinn talks about how, when we're in the shower, we can be thinking about anything but the shower and that's a suboptimal way to spend those precious minutes. He suggests stepping into the cubicle and leaving the to-do list outside. It's not a big chunk of the day to give to the opportunity to be present in your own head.

So, maybe try each day this week to step into the shower and focus on nothing apart from the sights, sounds and smells of your shower at that time.

Notice the pressure and temperature of the water. Feel where the water hits the back of your neck or place your face straight into it and feel the sensations.

Breathe and notice the sounds of the water changing with your position.

Smell that shower gel you normally ignore.

It's a highly effective and pleasant method of training your mind to become focused and grounded.

And you're doing it anyway. May as well do it mindfully and benefit in a new fresh way.

Another tip for busy people: when you're brushing your teeth, make that two minutes about nothing else but focus. Most electric brushes have a two-minute timer so there is no danger of you getting lost in time and being late for your shift. See if you can focus on nothing but the sounds, minty smells and feel of the brush. That's only four minutes a day which can make a massive difference. Not only will you have grounded yourself at the start and end of each day, you'll have great teeth!

Remember that you are doing all these exercises for you. You are taking back some control over your mind and you deserve this.

Language
See Part Six, Chapter 13 regarding the use of language.

Practise now using your internal chatter to say something positive to yourself. It can be literally anything. It can be that you've noticed that nothing awful happened during the night. Putting it into words is the exercise. Speak to yourself as you would speak to a friend you care about.

For example, when you find your keys in a random place as you're trying to rush out the door, instead of 'Ah, keys!', you could say 'OMG this is such a relief. I'm so chuffed I found them. This is great'.

This is not denying the fact that we have struggles or that the world has many simultaneous crises. It's simply actively noticing, more than we normally do, what is okay or even good.

You can have fun with this exercise. 'OMG this is such a relief. Delighted I found them. I love having a car. And a job, an interesting albeit a bit hectic one. This is a great start to the day...'. Even if it feels overly cheerful and disproportionate to the situation, it's a great exercise to do and then to notice what, if any, effect it has on your mood and on the vibes you're giving off to your colleagues.

Body
Sit up straight. Just for this exercise, notice and relax the shoulders. Place your feet on the ground and welcome the way it supports you always.

Breathe in and out. Notice what's not wrong with your health.

Some meditations to create a moment of positive emotional state using focus, language and body would be basic breath meditation, body scan meditation and hand on heart meditation (see Part Two). When busy at work, it takes a couple of seconds to think 'Focus, Language, Posture'. Then you could for example, take control of your focus and direct it towards one individual task for one patient, use language such as 'I'm doing well to take some charge of my present emotional state. This is good', and adjust your posture to have relaxed shoulders, no hunching over a screen and take a long deep breath.

Depersonalisation

Feeling like you're sleepwalking through life.
   Feeling like an onlooker to your life.
   Feeling like a zombie.
   Feeling like you're 'dead behind the eyes'.
   Feeling numb to other people's emotions (joy and sadness).
   This isn't necessarily a painful experience. Some people want to feel numb. Alcohol is often used to help us to feel a bit numb. Some antidepressants can cause this lack of feeling emotion too.

However, when being a zombie or an understudy in the story of your life makes you feel a void inside, it's called depersonalisation and many people don't want to feel like an android. Also, depersonalisation can affect those around us and our relationships with our loved ones.

A meditation to help us to connect or reconnect with others is the loving kindness meditation (see Part Two).

Disconnection from Purpose

> Can you live your life so deeply rooted in your purpose that even taking the bins out is meaningful?

So why do we go to work?

Close your eyes. Remember a time when you felt you had achieved something; maybe qualifying, placing your first IV catheter, finishing a race or sticking up for yourself against an antagonist.

Describe and write down the emotions you feel now as you remember it. Reconnect with those emotions and physical feelings. They were real. It happened. No matter how long ago or how different we feel now, it doesn't negate what we have achieved in the past. We've just moved on in life.

The exercise here is to notice what it feels like when we have a purpose in life. It drives us forward to achieve things.

Often, terminally ill people, on receiving their diagnosis, suddenly feel this huge sense of purpose. They make bucket lists which are inspirational, they fundraise and live longer than others who have a less positive, less purposeful attitude.

So, if we agree that having a purpose is part of the prevention of burnout, how do I find a purpose? My purpose?

Can I make a bucket list now? It needs to be achievable. Ideally a short-term purpose to start with.

The most important part of this exercise is to notice your connection with the purpose and how you feel as you're doing it and when you've finished it.

Needless to say, deciding to run a marathon for the first time is probably not the ideal first purpose; growing tomatoes, couch to 5 K park runs, reading this book and doing a meditation are all achievable, purposeful and can give rise to many previously ignored strong and positive emotions. Maybe you could connect right now with the purposeful reading of this text and think abut what you hope to achieve by reading it. This is purposeful, meaningful and can encourage you to find other drivers in your life too.

Summary of Strategies to Combat Burnout

When you're starting to feel emotionally exhausted.

- Reconnect to joy.
- Change your *focus* by grounding, and checking in with yourself a few times a day.
- Use *empowering language* and change your physiology with coherent breathing and progressive muscle relaxation, for good *posture*.

When you're feeling depersonalisation.

- Take your pulse.
- Reconnect with compassion towards others.
- Practice the loving kindness meditation.

When your *purpose* isn't clear,
when you're feeling unrewarded and unfulfilled by your job, reconnect to your purpose at work and observe what you actually *do* achieve even though you take it for granted as a minimum requirement.

Spend time with the other purposes outside work like putting the bins out and walking the dog.

Don't procrastinate. Try to do something small but purposeful each day, even if it's just watering the plants.

> *As long as you're breathing, there's more right with you than wrong with you.*
>
> Jon Kabat-Zinn

Being able to recognise burnout as it develops in yourself and others is life-saving knowledge. It is important because if we cannot take care of ourselves and recognise these symptoms, then we cannot take care of anyone else. We've already alluded to 'putting on your own oxygen mask before helping others with theirs'. It's not being selfish to look after yourself, it's altruistic if you then look after others when you're strong.

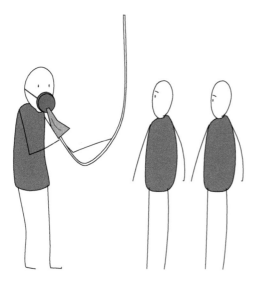

Neuroplasticity and Reversing Burnout

So we can recognise burnout in ourselves and we've applied a few strategies to combat the symptoms we can see to try to prevent the burnout progressing.

The good news is that the symptoms are reversible. The same mechanisms that led to those set points of normality changing negatively can also be harnessed to change those set points back to normal where the body can function more optimally. Those mechanisms are known as 'neuroplasticity' and epigenetics.

> Burnout is reversibe due to neuroplasticity.

In a nutshell, the way we are living our lives is changing our brain architecture (neuroplasticity) and how our genes are being expressed (epigenetics).

If we take a snapshot of your thoughts at any moment, you're often either rehashing the past or planning for the future. In fact, every time your mind wanders and you bring it back, it's like exercising a muscle. At first, you have to do many repetitions to build up that muscle. And every repetition (or noticing and bringing attention back) is a welcome chance to exercise that muscle and is something to be celebrated. With more practice, just as with more exercise, the 'muscle' becomes better and stronger.

Formal activities, e.g. meditation, and others which are informal, e.g. noticing all the tiny sights around you while walking, all help by bringing a mindful quality of attention into your daily life.

It's important to have a variety because different practices affect different areas in the brain. Mindfulness enables you to better apply the strategies to combat burnout.

The Evidence Base

Burnout is a pandemic issue and I am not talking about coronavirus. In the UK alone, burnout affects more than half of practising doctors (Locke 2020). Vets have four times the UK national rate of suicide which, according to several studies, is not merely because of the ease of access to euthanasia drugs. Suicide can be the result of burnout which, in turn, is the result of chronic unresolved stress.

Suicide, Burnout and Chronic Stress

Chronic unresolved stress is responsible for 60% of all NHS visits each year and is accounts for eight out of 10 of the leading causes of death in the UK (Schnall et al. 2009). So burnout is a problem, and veterinary surgeon and veterinary nurse burnout are monumental problems.

Recognising Burnout

If an older, overweight male collapses in the street while clutching their chest, what do you think is most likely to be happening to them? It's probably a heart attack but how did you know? You know because you can recognise the external signs of a heart attack. It is life threatening and because of this, everyone knows what to do next.

Similarly, being able to recognise burnout as it develops in yourself and others is life-saving knowledge. It is important because if we cannot take care of ourselves and recognise these symptoms, then we cannot take care of anyone else.

Mindfulness and Burnout

Many of us have our own self-care practices; we know that if we eat healthily, exercise regularly and sleep for eight hours each night we can manage stress better. But a lot of us do that and still reach the point of burnout.

Study after study shows that mindfulness practices and living mindfully tend to be the overarching ingredients that are missing when we mismanage stress. Mindfulness has over 50 years of research showing how it can affect neuroplasticity and reverse the changes in the mind and body caused by chronic unresolved stress (Hölzel et al. 2011). The American Mindfulness Research Association (https://goamra. org/publications/mindfulness-research-monthly) is a great place to discover all the high-quality research that has been done so far. The rest of this chapter will summarise a few of the outcomes of recent studies in three key areas: emotional, physical and mental health.

Emotional Health

Mindfulness has been shown to enhance focus and attention so that we are better able to begin and complete tasks (Norris et al. 2018). Even children who practise mindfulness do better at school, and we are starting to see curricula that incorporate mindfulness becoming more prevalent in UK schools.

Mindfulness also helps you to regulate your emotions so that emotional triggers do not aggravate you as much. This also means that your autonomic nervous system is not so easily hyperactivated so life's turbulence becomes more manageable day to day.

Mindfulness and meditation can also influence our compassion. A study was conducted on a group of people asking them to practise loving kindness meditation before they were shown pictures of strangers, while a second group did not practise this meditation before they were shown these pictures. The group that meditated beforehand attributed more positive qualities to those strangers than the group that did not meditate (Kok and Singer 2017).

What does that tell us about compassion? Compassion is a perception-based skill; it can be learnt and it can be lost.

Physical Health

With regard to the clinical outcomes of mindfulness research on physical health, studies have shown the following.

- Mindfulness reduces the risk of cardiovascular events and improves cardiovascular health (Loucks 2015).
- Mindfulness reduces chronic pain by as much as 60%, compared to opioids which reduce pain by only 15–30% (Zeidan and Vago 2016).

- Mindfulness can enhance the immune system post vaccination: a group of subjects that did mindfulness before receiving a flu vaccination mounted a more robust immune response than those who did not (Davidson et al. 2003).
- Mindfulness helps healing: in patients who had psoriasis and were undergoing light therapy, a study showed that they healed four times faster when they did mindfulness during their therapy than patients who just listened to relaxing music (Kabat-Zinn et al. 1998).

Mental Health

It has been shown that mindfulness can be curative for many mental health disorders, especially insomnia, anxiety and depression. Even in people who practised an eight-week intervention once without ever doing so again, studies could measure those positive changes three years down the line and still notice them.

Mindfulness also can slow down brain ageing. Long-term meditators in their 50s who practise mindfulness were seen to have brains that resemble those of 30 year olds on MRI scans. Mindfulness also appears to slow down genetic ageing by reducing the activity of an enzyme which shortens the DNA with age (Santarnecchi et al. 2021).

Mindfulness Mentality and Change

Inside the brain, what you focus on expands. We can look at your brain under an MRI scanner and discover whether you tend to live on the more depressive side of life or on the happier side of life. But the good news is that this mentality is not hard-wired; your brain architecture changes with every one of your experiences.

> Start your day with gratitude. Because what you focus on expands and becomes all you see.

So, maybe clinical research results in a well-respected, peer-reviewed publication will be the stimulus that starts you on your journey into mindfulness, or will provide you with the boost you need to take your practice to the next level. Hopefully mindfulness will provide you with the ability to improve your emotional, physical and mental health, thus enabling you implement the strategies that prevent, combat and reverse burnout. That may then change your life long term, who knows? Nothing is permanent, everything changes, and that is okay.

References

Davidson, R.J., Kabat-Zinn, J., Schumacher, J. et al. (2003). Alterations in brain and immune function produced by mindfulness meditation. *Psychosomatic Medicine* 65: 564–570.

Hölzel, B.K., Carmody, J., Vangel, M. et al. (2011). Mindfulness practice leads to increases in regional brain gray matter density. *Psychiatric Research* 191: 36–43.

Kabat-Zinn, J., Wheeler, E., Light, T. et al. (1998). Influence of a mindfulness meditation-based stress reduction intervention on rates of skin clearing in patients with moderate to severe psoriasis undergoing phototherapy (UVB) and photochemotherapy (PUVA). *Psychosomatic Medicine* 60: 625–632.

Kok, B.E. and Singer, T. (2017). Phenomenological fingerprints of four meditations: differential state changes in affect, mind-wandering, meta-cognition, and interoception before and after daily practice across 9 months of training. *Mindfulness* 8: 218–231.

Locke, T. (2020). Medscape UK Doctors' Burnout & Lifestyle Survey 2020. www.medscape.com

Loucks, E.B. (2015). Positive associations of dispositional mindfulness with cardiovascular health: the New England Family Study. *International Journal of Behavioral Medicine* 22: 540–550.

Norris, C.J., Creem, D., Hendler, R., and Kober, H. (2018). Brief mindfulness meditation improves attention in novices: evidence from ERPs and moderation by neuroticism. *Frontiers in Human Neuroscience* 12: 315.

Santarnecchi, E., Egiziano, E., D'Arista, S. et al. (2021). Mindfulness-based stress reduction training modulates striatal and cerebellar connectivity. *Journal of Neuroscience Research* 99 (5): 1236–1252.

Schnall, P.L., Dobson, M., Rosskam, E., and Elling, R.H. (2009). *Unhealthy Work: Causes, Consequences, Cures.* New York: Taylor and Francis.

Zeidan, F. and Vago, D. (2016). Mindfulness meditation-based pain relief: a mechanistic account. *Annals of the New York Academy of Sciences* 1373: 114–127.

Management and Mindfulness

- Mindfulness as an evidence-based tool to prevent stress, burnout and depersonalisation
- How do we promote mindfulness training in our practices?

Mindfulness as an Evidence-based Tool to Prevent Stress, Burnout and Depersonalisation

> Being proactive is better than reacting to burnout after it has damaged one's professional life or personal wellness.

Someone asks you what you do for a living. You tell them you're a vet or a vet nurse. Don't you find that people react with a lot of interest? Often with a degree of longing for our career as they always wanted to be a vet or nurse. And then the question 'What's the strangest animal you've ever treated?'. The general assumption is that we are living the dream career-wise.

There's a long queue of disappointed A-level students desperate to get onto a veterinary medicine course and countless numbers of students trying to do the veterinary nursing course. And yet there's a surprisingly long queue (42% of us) wanting out of the professions in some way or another. The older, jaded and disillusioned queue of vets and nurses never lets on to the younger, optimistic and naïve queue, and so the circle of irony continues uncontested and rarely mentioned.

Our job offers us the potential for tremendous personal and professional satisfaction. Few careers provide the opportunity to have such a profound effect on the lives of others and to derive meaning from work. To experience the joy of facilitating healing, and to help support those patients who can manage a good quality of life despite their medical diagnoses is a pleasure that often passes us by. Why?

Maybe we are focusing too much on what needs to be done next. Maybe we are disregarding our clinical successes as they don't need our attention any more and instead, we are on to solving the next case. Well, that's the way we work. It's often the way I work. We'd never get through the ops list if we spent our time basking in the glory of one case which went beautifully.

Is that mindful working? It isn't.

The avoidance of pausing to observe what is good at work and what is going well for us for fear that we might waste time is prevalent amongst many vets and nurses.

And yet if we take one minute to appreciate a case which is going well, however minor a case it may be, we might just find that *that* moment of mindful working contributes to better time management for the next few hours.

We have a responsibility to ourselves, to our colleagues and most importantly to our patients and their owners to manage the stressors unique to our career path, to determine the optimal balance of noticing the successes while being driven to treat the next patient with excellent concentration, and to nurture our personal wellness.

When we are stressed or even just mildly overwhelmed or flustered, we are less focused on the individual patient. That is not optimal care.

Morbidity and mortality reviews of surgical errors show that one of the main reasons for gross errors such as operating on the wrong limb, mistaking a patient's identity, performing the incorrect procedure (e.g. laparotomy to castrate a normal male) is that the vet was not focused. They were thinking of something else which was apparently more urgent. Basically, they were not being mindful. Mindfulness is not a luxury which vet and nurse teams with short ops lists partake in at their leisure. Mindful working is paramount if we are to perform to the best of our ability and thus avoid many of the errors which would drive us to join the queue to leave the professions.

A study by Lebares (2018) looked at burnout and stress among US surgery residents. Its findings ring true for many healthcare professionals and, I believe, very much so for veterinary professionals. Lebares noted the connection between the mental health of the practitioner (i.e. us) and how it affects patient outcomes. In other words, we do have a responsibility to be emotionally healthy if we are to practise good medicine and surgery. Mental wellbeing should not be a choice we can opt out of – it should be a job requirement.

> Mental wellbeing should not be a choice we can opt out of – it should be a job requirement.

Lebares examined burnout and the psychological characteristics that can contribute to burnout vulnerability and resilience in a group of surgical trainees. While we are not human surgeon trainees, there are many parallels between us and the doctors in the study.

Burnout was assessed with an abbreviated Maslach Burnout Inventory. Stress, anxiety, depression, resilience, mindfulness and alcohol use were assessed and analysed for prevalence. Truthfully, how many of these appear in your life?

- Stress?
- Anxiety?
- Resilience?
- Mindfulness?
- Alcohol?

Among the 566 surgical residents who participated in the survey, burnout was at a whopping 69%, equally driven by emotional exhaustion and depersonalisation. Depersonalisation involves a persistent or recurring feeling of being detached from one's body or mental processes. To some, it may feel like going through the motions, purposefully feeling as little as possible in order to get through the day.

Depression, suicidal ideation and anxiety were notably high across training levels, but improved with greater experience.

For the statisticians amongst us (even mental health studies use statistics), odds ratios (ORs) were used to determine the magnitude of presumed risk and resilience factors. I include the OR in brackets just to stress the differences between burnout and mindful working.

Higher burnout was associated with high stress (78), depression (48) and suicidal ideation (57). However, in contrast, Lebares found that **dispositional mindfulness** was associated with lower risk of stress (0.15), depression (0.26) and suicidal ideation (0.25). These figures are obviously vastly different.

> The case for mindfulness is so strong that for HR not to promote it as part of the workplace culture is to miss a real opportunity to optimise patient care by promoting clinician self-care.

This study unquestionably supports the potential of mindfulness training to promote resilience, decrease exhaustion and burnout and improve the standard of care we provide to our patients. Being proactive is better than reacting to burnout after it has damaged one's professional life.

How Do We Promote Mindfulness Training in Our Practices?

Have a mindfulness CPD day with a qualified mindfulness practitioner. This counts as RCVS CPD and is tax deductible.

Set up a mindfulness hub in your practice and employ the mindfulness practitioner to teach staff how to use it for mini-meditations.

Gift this book or any other book on mental wellbeing for veterinary professionals to your new staff, your existing staff. your new graduates and your managers. Make a book club meeting about it.

Reference

Lebares, C., Guvva, E., and Ascher, N. (2018). Burnout and stress among US surgery residents: psychological distress and resilience. *Journal of the American College of Surgeons* 226: 80–90.

Suicide in the Veterinary Professions

- The perfect storm in vets
- The neurobiology of suicide
- How do we increase our production of oxytocin?
- Understanding the steps towards suicide

What causes lethal emotional pain? What is it within our psyche that leads to such a high rate of dying by suicide?

While this chapter shows that access to means and its withdrawal can be the single most effective way of preventing suicide, preventing suicidal ideation amongst our colleagues in the veterinary professions cannot remain taboo.

> The millisecond my hands left the rail, it was instant regret.

Kevin Hines, one of the 2% of people who jumped from the Golden Gate Bridge and survived.

Interestingly, in his article 'Jumpers' in *Psychology Today* magazine, Steve Taylor talks of 29 other Golden Gate Bridge survivors who *all* said they instantly regretted their decisions to end their lives.

Ken Baldwin is one such 'jumper'. As soon as he let go, he knew he'd made a mistake. Despite all his years of contemplating suicide, he knew that he didn't want to die after all. As he describes it, 'I thought, what am I doing? This was the worst thing I could do in my life. I thought of my wife and daughter. I didn't want to die. I wanted to live'. He recalls realising that 'everything in my life that I'd thought was unfixable was totally fixable – except for having just jumped'.

Other jumpers say: 'I've changed my mind', 'This is a terrible mistake', 'How do I undo this?'.

Jumping from the Golden Gate Bridge in order to take your own life is so successful that it's fair to presume that those who do it are serious about suicide being the solution to their life's problems. So, these interviews have weight. Similarly, it's also safe to presume that many others who have actually been successful in killing themselves also regretted their actions after it was too late.

Suicide is not the solution. It doesn't fix anything. It only makes it worse for the loved ones left behind and for the person jumping for the last few seconds of their life.

Kevin Hines talks about the voices in his head compelling him to take his life. Like most people suffering from suicidality, he felt he was a burden to those close to him, he felt no sense of future and his internal voice told him there was an easy way out.

The most common diagnosis among those who die by suicide is manic depressive disorder.

So, what makes the thought of living so unbearable that dying is more favourable? What causes this lethal emotional pain?

In US adolescents, the second most common reason for death is suicide (www.childrenshospital.org). There are multiple factors driving them to it. In the UCL Millennial Cohort Study where 19 000 young people were interviewed in 2018–2019, 7% said they had attempted suicide by the time they had reached 17 years of age.

The Perfect Storm in Vets

Dr Eboni Webb, Doctor of Clinical Psychology from the Minnesota School of Professional Psychology, specialises in dialectical behaviour therapy (DBT). She says that her suicidal clients suffer from:

- emotional vulnerabilities, which can come from many sources but that their vulnerability is often biological
- chronic and consistent invalidation which exacerbates their emotional vulnerabilities
- an ongoing, reciprocal relationship between their emotional vulnerabilities and their environment.

Maybe this is why a perfect storm is created when vets who are emotionally vulnerable receive chronic criticism (sometimes our own internal chatter), are overwhelmed by their workload and work demands and have access to means in the unregulated, unmanned dangerous drugs cupboard.

The Neurobiology of Suicide

During 'intense, lethal emotional pain', cortisol is produced excessively by the hypothalamic-pituitary-adrenal (HPA) axis. This cortisol leads to dysfunction at different levels of the HPA axis and results in clogging of the corpus callosum connecting the left and right hemispheres of the brain (Suzuki et al. 2014).

Blood flow decreases to the prefrontal cortex (which is needed for reasoning) and to the non-dominant hemisphere. Blood flow increases to the heart and extremities and decreases to the gut where 70% of our serotonin is normally produced.

Adolescents are more vulnerable to stress because the prefrontal lobes, which are needed to manage life's normal ups and downs, take 25 years to develop fully. How inconvenient is that, given that we have so many ups and downs as teenagers?

So, the one part of the brain which could making living more appealing than death isn't even running at full strength when we're young. And when we've reached crisis point with cortisol production off the scale, it's barely perfused at all. Along with that, our gut serotonin, which may take the edge off our suicidality, is practically non-existent.

In those of us over 25, some have better functioning prefrontal cortices than others. That's not the only reason we choose to live, but it helps.

During the impulsive phase just prior to suicide, cortisol production goes through the roof. Cortisol is counteracted by oxytocin, amongst other things.

How Do We Increase Our Production of Oxytocin?

Self-harming is one method. Skin pain causes jumps in oxytocin, so cutting your arm or leg is very soothing and empowering. Self-harming is a very complex issue beyond the scope of this chapter.

Psychotherapeutic treatment aims to increase oxytocin without self-destructive or harmful problem behaviours. DBT is a type of talking therapy based on CBT which is used to help people suffering from very intense emotional pain.

It would be good to train oxytocin to be of service to us. Other self-soothe skills include breath work, mindful meditation and mindful living. If you have a partner or close friend, hugs, back rubs, massage, positive eye contact are helpful. All these seemingly touchy-feely activities are evidence based and lead to increased levels of oxytocin.

Understanding the Steps Towards Suicide

Knowing that from making the final decision to dying takes an average of only 5–10 minutes, how can we stop the action?

Conceptualising Suicide
Conceptualising suicide is where there is a breakdown in problem solving, a perception of having no options and of suicide being one's only means of exerting control over this intense emotional pain.

Suicidal Ideation
Thoughts of ending life or of not living are common in all of us from time to time.

Because suicidal ideation also functions as an emotion regulation strategy, it may not reflect a true desire to die or be a source of extreme distress to the person feeling it, because in a paradoxical way it serves to temporarily relieve anxiety by being a possibility if all else fails.

Planning for Suicide
This involves considering ways to end one's life and even 'practising' the method.

Intent to Follow Through
This is where ambivalence about suicide has tipped in the direction of following through, and the person begins to prepare for the event.

Research shows that the interval between deciding to act and attempting suicide can be as short as 5–10 minutes (Simon et al. 2001).

People tend *not* to substitute a different method when their chosen lethal method is unavailable (Mann et al. 2005). Therefore, means restriction is the most medically sound, evidence-based method of suicide prevention in a crisis (Daigle 2005).

Rosie Allister wrote a fantastic piece on suicide prevention in veterinary practices in *Veterinary Practice*: www.veterinary-practice.com/article/five-evidence-based-steps-for-suicide-prevention-in-veterinary-practices.

Furthermore, knowing that the critical danger period is a short-lived impulsive crisis, by means restriction at the time of the person's greatest risk, we provide them with the alternative which is to seek effective evidence-based interventions and the opportunity to do what so many other suicidal people wished they'd done – seek help.

> *No one's gonna know that I didn't want to die.*
>
> Kevin Hines

References

Daigle, M.S. (2005). Suicide prevention through means restriction: assessing the risk of substitution. A critical review and synthesis. *Accident; Analysis and Prevention* 37: 625–632.

Mann, J.J., Apter, A., Bertolote, J. et al. (2005). Suicide prevention strategies: a systematic review. *JAMA* 294: 2064–2074.

Simon, T.R., Swann, A.C., Powell, K.E. et al. (2001). Characteristics of impulsive suicide attempts and attempters. *SLTB* 32 (supp): 49–59.

Suzuki, A., Poon, L., Papadopoulos, A.S. et al. (2014). Long term effects of childhood trauma on cortisol stress reactivity in adulthood and relationship to the occurrence of depression. *Psychoneuroendocrinology* 50: 289–299.

Part 4

Therapy

Cognitive Behavioural Therapy

Cognitive behavioural therapy (CBT) doesn't negate your feelings. It doesn't brush aside the seriousness of the situation. However, it prevents us from 'awfulising' and making the situation worse. It helps us to get things in perspective in order that we may work effectively to solve problems.

The CBT model is a simple one, which encourages the examination of *thoughts* before they become *feelings* which would determine our *behaviours*.

We can't stop the way we've been thinking for years just at will. We can, however, develop *logical* reactions to those thoughts and learn to recognise thought patterns which are having a detrimental effect on our lives because they are giving rise to negative feelings and negative behaviours as if we have no control over them.

Rational Emotive Behavioural Therapy

Rational emotive behavioural therapy (REBT) is a type of CBT that aims to help a person challenge unhelpful thoughts in order to avoid negative reactions and behaviours.

REBT focuses attention on the present using mindfulness techniques, and helps us to develop a new way of thinking about events to prevent maladaptive behaviours and negative emotions.

It probably sounds a bit contradictory to the idea of acceptance of our emotions. The difference here is that if, through self-awareness (I know how I'm likely to feel in a given scenario), we can prepare for the thoughts and stop them in their tracks *before* they give rise to feelings which we ourselves have identified as irrational and unhelpful, then we can stop the spiralling of these feelings into actions and emotions which are hurting us.

For example, imagine I have a phobia of crossing the road because I believe that if I cross the road I will be hit by a car. And yet, I really want to be able to cross roads to pick my kids up from school, get to work, etc. So I decide that my phobia or intense fear is stopping me from achieving what I desire in order to have a satisfactory life.

My therapist will help me to decide if my goal of crossing the road is something I really want. Then they talk me through deciding whether

Mental Wellbeing and Positive Psychology for Veterinary Professionals: A Pre-emptive, Proactive and Solution-based Approach, First Edition. Laura Woodward.

my fear is rational or irrational. 'Irrational' is not considered to be a derogatory term in CBT. Yes, of course there is a chance that I will be run over if I cross the road. But how likely is it? Can I research the statistics? How many people get run over on that particular road each year compared to the number of people who cross it? Now how reasonable does the rational part of me feel that my fear is?

If I decide that I can accept those odds and take the risk because I feel it's minimal enough and also because I want to be able to do this for my quality of life, then I can relearn how to cross the road.

Role Play in REBT

Visualisation techniques are a good place to start. So, close your eyes and imagine yourself crossing the road, while observing safe crossing skills, Green Cross Code, etc. That will feel uncomfortable and probably cause anxiety. We've been here before in our chapter on allowing anxiety to be within us but not to rule us.

Once you have imagined it enough times and feel ready to move onto the next stage, it may be time to pretend you're crossing the road but only as you're walking across your living room floor.

By now, you're welcoming the feelings of anxiety. In fact, you want them to come to help you with this exercise. So they come and you 'cross' the road in your own house many times, being aware of your feelings and practising crossing safely at the same time.

The next stages are taken at your pace. Some people may take hours, others months. It depends on what fear you have and the type of person you are. No pace is better or worse than another.

You might approach the crossing a few times with a friend or alone. Then you might cross once or a dozen times alone or with someone. The idea is that, eventually, with your evaluation of the fears and their rationality, you are in charge.

This approach may help a person to achieve their goals and learn how to overcome adversity by addressing the underlying beliefs and thoughts that can lead to self-defeating or self-sabotaging actions. We use evidence based thinking to make decisions all the time at work. REBT appeals to vets and nurses often because of it's logical approaach. It's Rational. Using statistical analysis, and applying it to our fears is a very effective way of enabling us to decide if our concerns are rational or irrational. We don't have to necessarily dig into the reasons behind our sometimes irrational way of thinking to be able to tackle it.

Mindfulness-based Stress Reduction

- What is MBSR?
- Evidence base for MBSR
- Aims of MBSR

What is MBSR?

Mindfulness-based stress reduction (MBSR) is an eight-week evidence-based programme that offers secular, intensive mindfulness training to assist people with stress, anxiety, depression and pain.

Developed at the University of Massachusetts by Professor Jon Kabat-Zinn, MBSR uses a combination of meditation, body awareness and body scans, and exploration of patterns of behaviour, thinking, feeling and action.

Using the techniques in the How to Meditate section such as meditation, body scan and emotional intelligence to investigate with fresh eyes our self-awareness and self-regulation, under the guidance of a therapist, stress, anxiety and many of our workplace challenges can be stopped from ruling our headspace and our life.

MBSR is not just for veterinary professionals, our stressors are not just associated with our work. It can help anyone at any age in any job with any difficulty.

Jon Kabat-Zinn describes the MBSR programme in detail in his book *Full Catastrophe Living*. He describes how to use the power of focused awareness to meet life's inevitable challenges – one of the aims of this book you are holding. Knowing about MBSR and being aware of MBSR techniques used by your counsellor will already have a massive effect on your mental wellbeing.

The programme itself is intense. It is an eight-week workshop taught by certified trainers that entails weekly group meetings (2.5-hour classes) and a one-day retreat (seven-hour mindfulness practice) between sessions six and seven, homework (45 minutes daily), and instruction in three formal techniques: mindfulness meditation, body scanning and simple yoga postures (Kabat-Zinn 2013).

Group discussions and exploration are a central part of the programme. Group practice in Buddhism is called the Sangha. It may sound difficult but when you can chat about mindfulness with people who are in the same place as you physically and emotionally, it is so nourishing.

MBSR is based on non-judgement, non-striving, acceptance, letting go and other techniques you already know from the How to Meditate section.

Robert Sapolsky, a professor of biology and neurology at Stanford University, describes, ironically in a humorous way, the debilitating and life-threatening effects of stress on our bodies. His book *Why Zebras Don't Get Ulcers* tells us what we already know from physiology (Sapolsky 2004) and yet we tend to ignore it because that stuff happens to 'other people'.

Using MBSR to tackle our stress (and we all have at least a degree of underlying stress) will make us better citizens, happier in the workplace, nicer to be around as well as being around for longer, which we owe to our families.

> Waiting for the perfect time to start our stress management is our choice. However, we could instead just start.

Evidence Base for MBSR

Engaging in mindfulness meditation brings about significant reductions in psychological stress (Sharma and Rush 2014). MBSR prevents the associated physiological changes and biological clinical manifestations that happen as a result of psychological stress (Black and Slavich 2016).

MBSR has been shown to help separate the pain of arthritis from the emotional effects of chronic pain which we have explored in Part Three, Chapter 22 (DiRenzo et al. 2018), thus greatly reducing suffering from the pain.

Aims of MBSR

- Awareness of our mind.
- Awareness of our body.
- Awareness of stress and reduction of the physiological and the emotional burdens of stress.
- Exploration of uncomfortable emotions and physical pain in a safe environment to develop less emotional reactivity to them.

- Acceptance of life's challenges, changes and losses as natural parts of human existence.
- Non-judgement of our experiences.
- Learning to use our inner resources to live calmer, more joyful lives.

What if the feelings resulting from my thoughts are indeed rational and appropriate? Then other types of therapy may be useful.

References

Black, D.S. and Slavich, G.M. (2016). Mindfulness meditation and the immune system: a systematic review of randomized controlled trials. *Annals of the New York Academy of Sciences* 1373 (1): 13–24.

DiRenzo, D., Crespo-Bosque, M., Gould, N. et al. (2018). Systematic review and meta-analysis: mindfulness-based interventions for rheumatoid arthritis. *Current Rheumatology Reports* 20 (12): 75.

Kabat-Zinn, J. (2013). *Full Catastrophe Living: Using the Wisdom of Your Body and Mind to Face Stress, Pain, and Illness.* New York: Bantam Dell.

Sapolsky, R. (2004). *Why Zebras Don't Get Ulcers.* New York: Holt Paperbacks.

Sharma, M. and Rush, S.E. (2014). Mindfulness-based stress reduction as a stress management intervention for healthy individuals: a systematic review. *Journal of Evidence-Based Complementary and Alternative Medicine* 19 (4): 271–286.

Acceptance and Commitment Therapy

Acceptance and Commitment Therapy (ACT) is a type of therapy which encourages the patient to face their thoughts and feelings rather than trying to avoid them or shut them out. We have an instinct to control our experiences, but this instinct does not always serve us.

Instead of judging ourselves for having these feelings and deeming them as 'wrong', once we've established that our feelings are indeed rational, we face them and even embrace them as a natural part of the human existence.

Last week I heard a story about Picasso. Like a parable but not so ancient. Picasso was walking through the market when he was approached by a woman who recognised him as one of the greatest artists of all time. She asked him to draw something for her and he very kindly quickly sketched her something on a piece of paper. 'That will be thirty thousand dollars' he said.

'But' said the woman, 'it only took you thirty seconds to sketch this.'

'Actually' said Picasso, 'it took me thirty years!'

This story rang true with me because we so often fail to recognise the effort, perseverance and grit that go on behind the scenes in someone's life. Especially if they generally appear happy.

At work, we're so busy, we barely get time to grunt a 'hello' before launching into hospital rounds. And yet every person in that hospital has 'stuff' (a colloquial term for mental loads). Literally everyone has difficulties in their lives. It is the acceptance of these difficulties that allows us to actually function well.

Pushing our difficult emotions to one side is avoidance. We may appear to function on the outside. We might get through the ops list skillfully and greet our colleagues joyfully. But without acceptance of our 'stuff' and the multiple emotions it brings, all that skill and camaraderie won't bring us joy and peace of mind.

As therapists, we have so many qualifications and different methods of counselling in our toolboxes. One type of therapy does not fit all. Usually, my first meeting with a client is two or more hours long and designed to get a history and a real-time picture of their emotions and feelings, and

Mental Wellbeing and Positive Psychology for Veterinary Professionals: A Pre-emptive, Proactive and Solution-based Approach, First Edition. Laura Woodward.
© 2024 John Wiley & Sons Ltd. Published 2024 by John Wiley & Sons Ltd.

then we can dip into various modes of therapy before deciding which ones might be of help.

We have a plethora of therapies available, from CBT to MBSR, Internal Family Systems Therapy, empty chair therapy, person-centred therapy, the list is endless.

Acceptance and Commitment Therapy encourages the patient to face their thoughts and feelings rather than trying to avoid them or shut them out. Instead of judging ourselves for having these feelings and deeming them as 'wrong' or 'irrational', we face them and learn to accept them.

Buddhism talks a lot about human suffering. The Buddha taught the Four Noble Truths which I explained briefly in Part One, Chapter Four. Basically:

- There is suffering.
- There is a cause of suffering.
- There is an end to suffering.
- The way out is the Eightfold Path.

Doesn't sound very uplifting, right? By 'suffering', I imagine the Buddha meant the daily mental problems which are inevitable for us human beings. Animals don't have this mental angst going on in the background (usually), which is why they spend most of their day living in the moment, focusing on this walk, this toy, this food. And that brings them contentment and joy in everyday activities.

We are not spaniels, and that's okay.

If we can learn, using mindfulness techniques, to accept our emotions, then they may cause us pain but we will not be suffering.

Pain is inevitable. Suffering is optional. What does this mean? Basically, it is implausible to aim for a life without any hurdles or daily problems. However, the degree to which these hurdles hurt us is our choice.

> *Say you're running, and you think, 'Man, this hurts, I can't take it any more'. The 'hurt' part is an unavoidable reality, but whether or not you can stand any more is up to the runner himself.*
> Haruki Murakami, *What I Talk About When I Talk About Running*

ACT develops psychological flexibility and is a form of behavioural therapy that combines mindfulness skills with the practice of self-acceptance. When aiming to be more accepting of your thoughts and feelings, commitment plays a key role. In the case of ACT, you commit to facing the problem head on rather than avoiding your stresses.

So, the aim isn't to fix or change the stressors. Rather, it is to accept the emotions they bring non-judgementally, which defuses their hold over us.

As vets and nurses, we have so many stressors inside and outside the workplace. We're so busy, we can't even begin to list the stressors. They're all in that grey cloud hanging over our heads raining adrenaline into our brains.

It seems counterintuitive that stopping to look at and list the stressors might help us to be less stressed. Maybe try it just once.

A few decades ago, scientists conducted an experiment in the Arizona desert where they built 'Biosphere 2', a huge steel and glass enclosure with circulating purified air, purified water, nutrient-rich soil and abundant natural light. It provided the perfect climate for plants, insects and animals to flourish. All was well except for one thing: the trees, when they reached a certain height, would simply fall down despite the perfect conditions.

The scientists in Arizona were puzzled. As it turns out, trees grow strong and grow deep roots not just in search of water. Rather, it is because of winds pushing and pulling the trees in different directions, making life a bit more difficult. The trees respond to that hammering by the elements by becoming stronger, with thicker trunks and deeper roots.

So, the hurdles and suffering in our lives can be used as a way of becoming stronger, more resilient and wiser. And we can then be the people who turn up at work less phased by the enormous ops list and queue of clients snaking down the street. We've seen these storms before and got through them many times.

In the case of ACT, you commit to facing the problem head on rather than avoiding your stresses. Imagine committing to actions that help you facilitate your experience and embrace any challenge.

ACT is based on the concept that pain is a natural and inevitable condition for humans. We have an instinct to control our experiences, but this instinct does not always serve us.

The six core processes of ACT guide patients through therapy.

- Acceptance
- Cognitive defusion

- Being present
- Self as context
- Values
- Committed action

Acceptance is an alternative to our instinct to avoid thinking about negative (or potentially negative) experiences. It is the active choice to allow unpleasant experiences to exist, without trying to deny or change them.

Cognitive defusion refers to techniques intended to change how an individual reacts to their thoughts and feelings. ACT does not intend to limit our exposure to negative experiences, but rather to face them and come out the other side with a decreased fixation on these experiences.

Being present is the practice of being aware of the present moment, without judging the experience. We've learnt this skill in previous chapters.

Self as context is the idea that an individual is not simply the sum of their experiences, thoughts or emotions. *We are not only what happens to us. We are the ones experiencing what happens to us.*

Values in this context are the qualities we choose to work towards in any given moment. In the veterinary world, these may be patience, resilience, calmness, insightfulness, etc.

Finally, ACT aims to help patients *commit to actions* that will assist in their long-term goals and live a life consistent with their values. Positive behaviour changes cannot occur without awareness of how a given behaviour affects us.

It's this commitment to mental wellbeing which goes on behind the scenes of those happy, carefree cheerful colleagues you meet. You know, the person who always has time for you and a hug for you. The receptionist who never gets fazed by the clients, the surgeon who can deal with complications with an aura of calm, the ECC nurse who hits the artery every time and calculates CRI rates like a ninja.

Just like Picasso made superhuman efforts to become an amazing artist, the effort put into being happy can be massive. ACT is just one of the many exciting tools at our disposal.

> Meditation changes the mind's capacity to see life as it is and accept it; not by beating it into submission, but by making it clear that acceptance is a choice.

Acceptance and Commitment Therapy and Cancer

Acceptance and commitment therapy (ACT) is widely used by therapists for the anxiety that cancer survivors experience on 're-entry'. Cancer survivors may experience uncertainty about the meaning and purpose of their lives following cancer, triggering anxiety. Additionally, they may worry: 'Does this symptom mean that my cancer is back?', 'How can I live knowing that my cancer might return?' and 'Now that treatment is over, why I am not back to normal?'. Fear of cancer recurrence figures prominently, yet the focus of anxiety extends beyond just that.

Moreover, anxiety often persists for a decade or more after cancer treatment, representing the largest mental health difference between long-term cancer survivors and community controls.

We have discussed acceptance before. In a nutshell, *acceptance* is allowing ourselves to feel any emotion we are feeling non-judgementally. One at a time, you can identify what that emotion is, give it a name, feel the physical effects of that emotion, look it in the eye and notice that it's present. That's the opposite of shutting those feelings in a box only for them to come back another day and grab us unawares.

Commitment is committing to what we want to do as a result of each emotion we are feeling. Internally, that might be deciding to live with it and even 'befriend' it. Alternatively, it may be deciding to let it go for now or for longer. Neither is 'right' nor 'wrong'. Externally, we may decide on physical actions, e.g. do I want to shout? Do I want to give a loud sigh? Do I want to run away? Do I want to just not reply to messages? Do I want to make plans to meet a friend and then cancel at the last minute because I just can't face it?

Making these decisions consciously is helpful because it means that each reaction is not just us running on autopilot, it's us being self-regulated. The spin-off of good self-regulation is happier, more content people with positive interactions with others.

ACT promotes forms of coping that predict positive psychosocial outcomes among cancer survivors: actively accepting cancer-related distress, reducing cancer-related avoidance, clarifying personal values and committing to meaningful behavioural change.

Mental Wellbeing and Positive Psychology for Veterinary Professionals: A Pre-emptive, Proactive and Solution-based Approach, First Edition. Laura Woodward.
© 2024 John Wiley & Sons Ltd. Published 2024 by John Wiley & Sons Ltd.

ACT allows for, rather than minimises, the distress of cancer and fear of recurrence – an approach that may authentically validate the fears of re-entry phase survivors, many of whom live with the real possibility of relapse and early mortality. Thus, ACT may help cancer survivors increase their capacity to live meaningfully and effectively even with persistent side-effects and uncertainty about the future. One of the aims of ACT is to help cancer patients and cancer survivors begin to 'live' again alongside depressed feelings and depressogenic thoughts.

I am in awe of cancer survivors who show any indication that they are accepting of these anxieties. Often, society and even the closest of family members are so joyful for the cancer survivor when they come to the end of their treatment, and are given a clean bill of health, that the survivor feels totally alienated from those they are closest to. At a venue where I counsel cancer survivors and cancer patients, I will often spend time with a survivor who has the long wished-for discharge note from their oncologist as they emerge from the rigorous schedule of months or years of appointments and treatment. The champagne corks are popping, balloons are everywhere and the survivor feels more alone than ever. Their family is celebrating but their support network has just evaporated as they are discharged from the only group of people who can truly understand how they feel. Some clients have said that they would choose to not be in remission or cured of their cancer rather than face this 're-entry'.

The expectation to celebrate and share in the optimism of your loved ones is often just too great for the cancer survivor.

Many regulars who come to this cancer support centre are in remission or even considered cured after five years of being cancer free. And yet, they feel more in common with their friends here then they do with the cancer-free population outside the door.

The strength and courage which some cancer survivors need when getting back to 'normality' are often greater than the strength they needed to get through their treatment.

Animal-assisted Therapies

- Communication
- Collaboration
- Respect

Animal-assisted therapies are different from other interventions and can overcome the limitations of human-to-human interaction as they don't rely on the use of talking and listening as a medium for change.

Equine psychotherapy is one such intervention. Equine-assisted psychotherapy (EAP) comprises a collaborative effort between a licensed therapist and a horse professional working with clients to address treatment goals.

> The purpose of the present Australian-based qualitative study was to examine EAP facilitators' perspectives on the biopsychosocial benefits and therapeutic outcomes of EAP for adolescents experiencing depression and/or anxiety. The findings suggest a range of improvements within adolescent clients, including increases in confidence, self-esteem and assertiveness, as well as a decrease in undesirable behaviours. The effectiveness of the therapy was thought to be due to the experiential nature of involving horses in therapy.
>
> *Wilson et al. (2017)*

The following quote regarding EAP appeared in 2017 (Wilson et al. 2017): 'The lack of understanding in the wider community about EAP was seen as a barrier to recognition and acceptance of EAP as a valid therapeutic intervention'

Most of us appreciate how effective pets-as-therapy (PAT) dogs are at lifting the mood of residents of care homes, and helping young people with chronic medical conditions who require long-term care away from home. In our very busy hospital, the staff will regularly pause to stick our noses into the kennel of a patient who wants to be stroked as much as we want to stroke them. It's the perk of the job.

Mental Wellbeing and Positive Psychology for Veterinary Professionals: A Pre-emptive, Proactive and Solution-based Approach, First Edition. Laura Woodward.
© 2024 John Wiley & Sons Ltd. Published 2024 by John Wiley & Sons Ltd.

In registered cat-friendly practices, the cat ward is a haven where music plays at the same BPM as a relaxed cat, blankets are plentiful and sprayed with pheromones, the patients have somewhere to perch and somewhere to hide and the sound of purring is everywhere. These patients often need a chin rub and some eye contact before they will touch their breakfast. It is interesting that, with the right level of calm and mutual respect between nurses and cats, the cats don't resent gentle handling, they co-operate with being examined and often the purring continues despite the placement of IV catheters, taking of blood and other unpleasant impositions.

As psychotherapists, we have a whole world of therapeutic interventions at our disposal. However, animal-assisted interventions (AAIs) are often left unused due to lack of understanding.

As vets and nurses, we are perfectly placed to understand, promote and benefit from AAIs and we make use of animal therapy subconsciously every day. Maybe we have no concerns which we feel warrant intervention or therapy. And yet subconsciously, we receive this therapy in spite of our perception that our problems don't reach the threshold of requiring it.

So what came first? Not needing therapy? Or the therapy we get every time we have a human–animal interaction, which may preclude our need for other therapy?

> Animal-assisted interventions are different from other interventions and can overcome the limitations of human-to-human interaction as they don't rely on the use of talking and listening as a medium for change.

There are many equine psychotherapy centres around the UK. One which I visited is called Strength and Learning Through Horses (SLTH) based in north London. At present, SLTH helps 500 people per year with a huge waiting list. However, they aim to help 750 per year. I have included quotes from some of the people who attend this centre.

Naïvely, when I visited SLTH, I had expected a herd of bomb-proof Thelwell ponies who would be available for brushing and feeding. I knew that placing one's hand on the horse's thorax to feel the heartbeat and breathing as the horse breathes can be a beautiful mindfulness practice. This, however, is not a herd of docile, jaded little ponies.

Trauma and PTSD, neglect and mistreatment, abuse, inability to trust others, anxiety, fear, anger, loneliness. This may look like a list of human predicaments treated at the centre, but they are just some of the past experiences and present realities of the beautiful horses at SLTH.

The horses vary in size, age and history. They are magnificent and powerful, some of whom are ex racing thoroughbreds (i.e. 'failures', 'rejects').

This was so humbling. As soon as I entered, a massive grey mare greeted me. I went to stroke her. She mistrusted me instantly even though I never did her wrong – she bared her teeth and told me to get lost, which I respected. I soon realised that I have much to learn.

So similar to when I meet some teenagers for our first therapeutic session: distrusting, cautious, closed off, angry. At least this horse communicated all of this, something which people often find hard to do.

And therein lies the beauty of equine therapy. Horses often communicate far more clearly than humans. We like to think of ourselves as eloquent and communicative but, with just facial and body language, a horse is so honest and truthful, and the young people who come to SLTH appreciate this. It may be something they have never experienced before.

> I can't even explain how 'unfed up' I am here.

Here, whatever your age, gender, race or nationality, the horse is non-judgemental. If you made a mistake at work, let your family down or didn't turn up for your GCSEs, the horse doesn't hold it against you.

You can be autistic, bipolar or have a history of abuse. The horse will not judge you for that. The horse is not here to 'fix' you – that would be judging you as 'wrong'.

> I have more resilience than I thought, and I am not a bad person. I actually have potential and have a future. Nothing has helped my confidence more than this place.

Communication

The horse is here to help you to communicate with them, with yourself and with others. There is nothing to compare with the moments when you and your horse are looking at each other, sussing each other out through observing breath, body language, facial expressions and heart rates of both of you.

It is true mindfulness being present in those moments, as well as being so much more than just a mindfulness practice.

There is no rush here, unlike the ticking clock in the counsellor's room where the therapist 'hour' is 50 minutes long. You cannot rush an interaction with a horse. It's physically dangerous and defeats the object of communication.

Matt, the horse professional, explained that often people will confide in their horse once the mutual trust, albeit it fragile and temporary, has been established. Matt and the psychotherapist back away at these times to allow for privacy.

The results are remarkable. This is a cohort of very troubled people for whom traditional therapies and medications often haven't helped. At SLTH, they don't cherry pick their clients. They take on new people based on whose need is the greatest. That in itself shows such courage. A characteristic we need if we are to be effective therapists.

> This gives me the motivation to get through the week. My anxiety is so much less when I am here.

Collaboration

Matt also explained about collaboration. Many of the young people who have therapy at SLTH have been excluded from school or from society in general. They may spend their free time in a virtual world online or just be unable to interact effectively with others because of lack of role models, autism, ADHD or any other cause.

Group therapy here involves small groups coming from many different walks of life. Again, gender, race and your history are accepted in a non-judgemental setting.

Sometimes there may be a task set for the young people. There is no horse riding here but the horses need to have a halter and rein placed to be led somewhere. This could be the task set for a group of three people, for example: go into the stable of that fearful huge mare, place a halter on her and lead her to the field.

Matt sees people unused to teamwork or co-operation use their various skills to attempt this task. Everyone is good at something. Maybe one person knows their way around a halter, maybe another has established a connection with this horse already and understands their need for slow movements, or non-judgementally accepts the horse's fear of loud talking. Perhaps the third person can make decisions and bring the group together, assigning talents to tasks.

Respect

How Matt and the staff treat the horses with respect and non-judgement is a thing of beauty. There is no mastering of unruly behaviour here.

If a horse needs space, they get it. Routines are not rigid because otherwise a slight routine change could be unsettling to a vulnerable horse who has become reliant on a routine for security. The horses are allowed to graze on the herbs and plants of their choosing (so long as they are safe), listening to their body's needs. Decreased stabling and less rugging up allow the horses to be more at one with their natural surroundings.

I've seen a lot of horses at riding schools in my time. However, I am very far from being knowledgeable about horses and horse behaviours. What I do remember from my past is seeing lots of crib biting, weaving, kicking and biting and finally submission to the spurs and crops. Here, there was no stereotypical behaviour to be seen, just behaviours. Despite their traumatic stories, these horses are now as lucky to be here as are the young people they assist.

Reference

Wilson, K., Buultjens, M., Monfries, M., and Karimi, L. (2017). Equine-assisted psychotherapy for adolescents experiencing depression and/or anxiety: a therapist's perspective. *Clinical Child Psychology and Psychiatry* 22 (1): 16–33.

Part 5

Case Studies

Introduction: The Counselling Process

Therapy: it's a mystery until you do it. We have the numbers to phone, the recommendations from the internet, lists of counsellors available for differing difficulties using a massive variety of methods which we know nothing about.

So how do you choose your therapist? There may be scores of CVs of therapists local to you with accompanying photos of kind-looking people. You look, try to narrow it down and then often it's left on the back burner because it's impossible to know who to open up to about your vulnerabilities, difficulties and backstory. Counsellors can use different types of talking therapies, CBT, MBSR etc. Psychotherapists do the same and can also prescribe treatments. Psychiatrists generally diagnose and treat psychopathologies eg., schizophrenia, manic depression etc.

I can't tell you who is best for you, but a counsellor is a good person to start with. Sometimes, you won't make a connection with the first therapist you meet. That does not mean that therapy isn't going to help you. It means you might need to look around a bit more.

Sometimes, you might work brilliantly with a therapist but after a while, you have gleaned as much from that therapeutic relationship as you can, and you move to someone who will help you further. It can be quite exciting.

> Making the call to make an appointment with a therapist is *not* an admission of failure or a sign that you are broken or weak.

It takes enormous courage to phone a random stranger and tell them that you need their help. This isn't ordering an Uber. It's so much more, and your stomach will churn while making the call.

I admire every one of my clients for filling in that contact form and then turning up.

Therapy should be seen as not just for when we are in crisis. It can be maintenance, like a car service, it can be a treat like a back massage.

I look on therapy as CPD for our mental wellbeing. Indeed, it is claimable as CPD and you can get tax relief on it. So I'm not alone in seeing therapy as an education.

Mental Wellbeing and Positive Psychology for Veterinary Professionals: A Pre-emptive, Proactive and Solution-based Approach, First Edition. Laura Woodward.
© 2024 John Wiley & Sons Ltd. Published 2024 by John Wiley & Sons Ltd.

Once you fill in the contact form or make the call, the usual process is for the therapist to arrange a brief phone call appointment to learn a bit about your difficulties and you can both decide if you'd like to start working together after that.

Once you've thought about it and decided to give it a go, an appointment is made. Then you've done it. All you have to do is turn up.

Most people wonder 'What will I talk about? I don't know where to start'. That's not your job, it's the counsellor's job.

In the first therapy session, the counsellor explains confidentiality. We are ethically bound by our accredited organisations to ensure complete confidentiality unless we feel you are a danger to yourself or to others. If we are concerned that you are going to harm someone else or yourself, we will ask you to contact your GP along with us. This is rarely needed.

Even if you arrange counselling through your practice and they pay for it, we are ethically bound to keep this complete confidentiality. Yes, we can send the practice an invoice, but we don't disclose anything, not even the dates you attended therapy.

The 'therapist hour' is 50 minutes long usually. This is because before and after your session, we need to make notes, think about you, and prepare for your next session.

Also, you will be asked not to turn up early because we don't want one client bumping into another on their way in and out of their sessions.

Some therapists prefer to allow the session to take as long as it takes and indeed some sessions can go on for hours.

In any case, it is the therapist's job to bring the session to a conclusion and then to an end.

Sometimes you will be asked to do some homework after a session, other times you won't.

Most therapists book clients into blocks of six, hour-long weekly appointments as a starting point.

Be prepared to be exhausted and thirsty after a productive session.

The people in the following case studies are happy to share their stories to help others. All names and several details have been changed to protect their anonymity. Although you might not be in exactly the same situation as the client, you may have many similarities.

These are descriptions of counselling sessions which took place. They are not verbatim reports but a summary of what happened.

Ann (A New Graduate Vet)

- First session
- Second session
- Third session
- Summary

Ann is six months into her first job as a vet. She contacted me for help because she was feeling overwhelming anxiety and felt she couldn't admit this to anyone at work for fear the team would think she was weak or 'not up to the job'.

Her home life has suffered as a result. She goes to work five or six days a week, comes home exhausted and stressed, eats and goes to bed. She can't sleep well because she is thinking about cases all night. The next day, she repeats the cycle of work, stress, eat and go to bed.

On her days off, she is irritable and just wants to be alone. She feels too exhausted to go out and socialise. She is getting no joy from anything outside work which she used to enjoy. She tries to go to the gym but even though she has some time for this, she doesn't have the energy or motivation any more.

First Session

When we first meet in my counselling room, Ann is pleasant but her body language is quite shut off. It's difficult to speak to someone in the veterinary world about work difficulties for fear of being judged. However, Ann feels that a counsellor who is a vet will understand her difficulties so much more than another counsellor.

Once I explain that everything which is said between us is always kept completely confidential and that I will only ever contact anyone regarding her story if I feel she is a grave danger to herself or to others, she relaxes into the sofa and takes a cushion onto her lap to hold.

I refer back to her email saying that she is feeling overwhelming anxiety at work and I ask her to explain what that feels like.

Mental Wellbeing and Positive Psychology for Veterinary Professionals: A Pre-emptive, Proactive and Solution-based Approach, First Edition. Laura Woodward.
© 2024 John Wiley & Sons Ltd. Published 2024 by John Wiley & Sons Ltd.

Ann has always been an A* student since as long as she can remember. Her younger sister is more arty than academic and struggled to have a good relationship with her parents, often going out on a bender and sleeping around. Ann was seen as the stable one, the golden child. She says she doesn't like this pressure from home to always succeed.

At university, Ann loved the course, loved seeing practice and the rotations and she wants to be a specialist surgeon someday.

At work, Ann says she is super nice to everyone. She greets the nurses and vets and knows everyone's name. The vets say 'Hi' but are always running around this busy practice.

People trust her to get on with her cases and to ask for help if she needs it. While this is a compliment, Ann says it actually pressures her into not asking for help.

I ask why. Ann stops to think for a little while and stares at the ceiling.

She feels that everyone expects her to succeed as she has always done. She's never needed help or guidance before and doesn't know how to ask for this.

I wonder how she would put it into words and I ask her to practise now how to ask a senior vet for help with a case.

Ann struggles to find words she is comfortable with.

Pause.

I ask, 'Can you describe what that discomfort feels like physically?' Ann describes a lump in her throat, she can feel her heart rate increase, a bit of a lurch in her stomach, her cheeks are flushed, her face looks full of tension. These are unpleasant physical feelings.

Ann finds these physical manifestations of stress so unpleasant, she would rather avoid them than ask a senior vet a question.

I wonder if the fear of feeling anxious is causing more anxiety in Ann. She agrees.

I ask Ann if she has learnt to meditate.

She hasn't.

So I teach her the first basic meditation to help to clear her mind so that we can work with this fear of anxiety.

We use a body scan meditation to relax Ann and then we try to focus on just the breath for a 15-minute meditation together.

I ask Ann to open her eyes and tell me how that felt. She takes a deep breath and says she found it deeply relaxing. It was the first time she had ever tried to meditate.

She found the guided body scan meditation quite easy and enjoyable. She found focusing on just the breath very hard. Her mind kept wandering and it was nearly impossible to stop it.

I explain that that is completely normal, for the first few times at least. Even monks have days when they struggle to focus on nothingness.

Every time her mind wanders away from the present or from her breath and she recognises it, that is a win. It's like exercising a muscle – it's going to take time and effort to get stronger and better at it.

Now I ask Ann to do a difficult exercise.

With her eyes closed, I ask her to put her hand on her neck and notice her breath, her chest rising and falling as well as her heart rate. She is relaxed and happy to do this.

Then I ask her to imagine she is having real difficulty with a case and needs to ask for help. I suggest a bitch spay bleeding. Then I ask her to describe the physical feelings.

She says her heart rate has rocketed, her jugular pulse is pounding, her breathing through her nostrils is noisy and rapid, she feels nauseous and like she may throw up.

We sit with those physical feelings for a while.

I ask her to decide on the words she is going to use to ask for help, all the while feeling sick and anxious. She comes up with the sentence 'I have a real problem with this spay and she's bleeding; please could you scrub in?'.

I ask her the emotional effects of saying this. Her heart rate is still through the roof and I can see her face is screwed up into a scowl. Her shoulders are raised up and rigid.

She pauses for a long time and then says 'I feel shameful. I have failed'.

We then spend some time just breathing, focusing on the breath and noticing her heart rate decrease again. She slowly relaxes her body a bit and sinks back into the sofa.

I ask her to only open her eyes when her breathing and pulse and stomach have returned to normal. It takes a minute or so.

When Ann opens her eyes, I ask her how she feels now. She says she feels relaxed again but that the exercise was really unpleasant.

In the counselling process when we feel that the client is ready, often we will 'challenge' them. This is not to alienate them but rather it is a way of teaching them that it's okay to challenge your own thought processes and beliefs. Sometimes, if we feel that our security in life is because of our steadfast way of thinking and doing, we don't want to challenge it or ever consider doing things differently. Especially if we are high achievers, we are reluctant to change anything in case our success falls apart. This fear of failure can spill into fear of changing anything in case it all suddenly goes wrong.

Using CBT helps to see where thoughts give rise to feelings which give rise to behaviours. In this case, recognising that if Ann asked for help, she knew she would feel ashamed and therefore chose the unhelpful (and possibly dangerous) behaviour of forging ahead unaided, we challenged this cycle together.

Also, using REBT, we challenged the preconception (or misconception, as Ann decided it was) that if I ask for help, everyone will presume I'm incompetent. After some thought, Ann put the risk of that as 'quite unlikely'.

So my challenge to Ann for this session is: You felt this anxiety, it is unpleasant for sure, but now that you've decided it's quite unlikely that everyone will think you're useless, could you accept these unpleasant physical feelings in return for being able to function in the workplace? Especially as you know that they are transient, physical sensations and you can make them move on afterwards with a simple breathing exercise.

Ann pauses for a while and then smiles. She says it's like a mini epiphany. That anxiety, while unpleasant, does not need to be avoided at all costs and certainly shouldn't be avoided if it's going to hold her back from her goals.

Acceptance

Unlike many average B or C students, Ann hadn't realised that many of us feel anxiety before GCSE exams or even end-of-term tests. We become so used to these feelings and physical sensations that we don't question them. We don't change our lives to avoid them at all costs even to the detriment of our careers. Feeling anxiety is a part of life. If you feel it, you are alive.

Ann's homework for that week was as follows.

1) Make time each morning for 20 minutes to do a body scan meditation and a breath meditation. Get up earlier and set an alarm for 20 minutes.

2) Role play asking for help. Observe the physical and emotional feelings.
3) Challenge the thought that everyone will think a certain way.
4) Practise asking for an opinion on at least two cases each day whether you need the help or not.
5) At work, when you feel an episode of anxiety, take a few moments to close your eyes and get in touch with your body. Name the feelings and the physical sensations. Focus one by one on the heart rate, the breathing rate, the stomach, the throat and try to accept that it's present, it's transient and it's expected.

Second Session

A week later Ann returned. She was finding the exercises easy some days and harder other days but was making a huge effort to do them diligently, which is in her nature. She was asking for help every day and sometimes framing it as simply a case discussion.

I wondered if it might be a good exercise to start a system of hospital rounds each day to discuss cases amongst the vets and nurses in the team. This is a great way to exchange ideas, improve quality of care and bond team mates together. It also teaches us not only to own our mistakes but to recognise our victories.

Ann, like many of us, rarely took any time to focus on what went right. She was too busy focusing on what went wrong or could go wrong.

I ask if she could try to establish the rounds and to make sure the cases which went right, even if just a cat castrate, could be discussed in a bit of detail so that the team as a whole could notice the positive cases. She agrees this would be a good exercise.

I probe a bit deeper this session about her family and background. I ask her if she had discussed these anxiety attacks with her family. She hadn't.

I ask if she wanted to tell them about it.

She is very relaxed in this session and happy and eager to chat. She tells me that she had this fear of letting her parents down especially as she was the golden child. They are so proud of her and boast to their friends about her which she finds embarrassing.

I ask her what she thinks their reaction would be if she opened up to them about work. She says she would rather pretend to them that all was well and 'leave them in their proud bubble' than tell them. She doesn't feel that telling them would achieve anything helpful, and that she would rather handle it independently of them.

I respect her wishes.

I ask her how her week has been at work apart from the exercises.

Ann's eyes light up whenever she talks about work. She's had a few great cases which went really well and she is taking the time and making the effort to recognise that they went well. That is bringing her more job satisfaction than she has had previously.

However, she has one case she can't get out of her mind. It was a stitch-up of a flank wound in a dog after a laceration on barbed wire.

She had asked for supervision from one of the vets and she's surprised at how easily already she can do this. She feels asking for assistance brings so little anxiety now compared to the anxiety associated with the prospect of this big stitch-up. The laceration was huge although only an hour old.

With all the appropriate care, Ann completed this stitch-up herself but it had taken her two hours.

I ask why she used the word 'but'. Again, Ann pauses and looks at the ceiling. It's always a good sign that the client is really thinking about the question and their answer.

She says it's because taking a long time for a simple procedure is 'failing' in some way.

I say nothing. Then Ann says that of course it's not failing. It's just being a new grad. She sutured the wound up which was 'succeeding' and not 'failing' because it took two hours.

I ask her if it's possible to look at things in two different ways. For example, taking two hours to compete a stitch-up can indeed be seen as failure by some and as a success by others. Could she choose which way to look at it if she took the time and made the effort? Ann agrees that this is a good strategy.

Then she says 'I succeeded in suturing that enormous wound up'.

She smiles.

Then she says that although she was doing all the mind clearing exercises we had practised, she kept waking up, or half walking up, during the night thinking about the dog. In her half-asleep mind, the wound broke down. Every time she closed her eyes, all she could see was a large flap of skin hanging down off this dog's side.

She is exhausted.

At the three-day check, Ann's anxiety has returned big time. For hours before the dog's appointment, she is presuming the worst. She can't express this to anyone and she's forgotten our anxiety-reducing meditation.

Awfulising

She's still pleasant to everyone and nobody knows the horrors going through her mind but her.

At the appointment, the wound check is good. The owners are compliant, the dog is bright and happy, the wound looks 'surprisingly okay' she says.

I ask Ann how she feels about it now. She sighs and says that she still feels that wound breakdown is inevitable and that nobody realises it but her. I ask her why she feels its 'inevitable'. She answers 'Because I've never done one before'.

We pause.

CBT talks about looking at our thoughts before they become feelings and deciding if they are rational or irrational, amongst many other things.

I ask Ann if all first-time stitch-ups break down, and if so, why? Ann recognises she is being challenged by me again.

We both know the answer.

Her thoughts, exacerbated by her nightmares, had become feelings and real beliefs that this wound was doomed to fail simply because it was her first one.

And yet, although this wound may very well break down, there will be a reason and it's unlikely it will be due to it being Ann's first stitch-up. There would be a clinical reason, possibly connected to inexperience but unlikely given the close supervision by an experienced surgeon she had been lucky to have looking over her shoulder.

Homework

Establish hospital rounds for a certain time each day and remember to notice what went right.

In ongoing cases, or prior to taking on cases, try to be clinical, evidence based and rational in deciding the prognosis.

When feeling low in confidence with a case, put it into words and express it to someone more experienced in that field. Not only are you showing yourself that you are human and that you are inexperienced (which is a fact), it's better for any case to have two minds on it than just one. Also, by expressing your fallibility, you are admitting to everyone that you still need guidance even though you look super-confident on the outside.

It's easy to forget what it's like to be a new grad unless the new grads remind us.

Third Session

At the start of the session, Ann is eager and excited to let me know that she has started hospital rounds at her practice. It's in the early stages at the moment and it's hard to get some of the vets to stop what they're doing to be present at rounds. She finds that everyone is agreed that it's a good thing and she's very proud she's taken this action.

A few of the nurses have expressed their appreciation that they are being included in group clinical discussions rather than being kept on the periphery as before, and Ann agrees that this has indeed bonded the team and already increased quality of care a lot even in just one week.

I ask her if she has managed to focus on what's gone right. She's finding this difficult because she's so busy, but recognises that this is a good idea and can be massively effective on her mood when she does it.

I ask her how her meditation practice is going. She is setting her alarm for 20 minutes earlier than normal every morning as well as leaving her normal alarm set so that she has literally 'created time' for meditation.

She is doing the body scan and breath meditation every morning. Sometimes this takes up the whole 20 minutes, and sometimes she tries to look at the cases she is anxious about and embrace that anxiety rather than try to shut it out.

I ask her how this is affecting her anxiety levels at work. Ann says it has changed her work life 'a full 180 degrees from terror to pleasure in the space of two weeks'.

I ask her about the dog stitch-up.

This time Ann tells me the dog's name and about his cheerful excitable personality. She stops, smiles and notes that this is the first time she has seen the dog as a whole dog instead of a piece of skin.

I ask her about this dog's owners and what they are like. Ann hasn't had the headspace to think about them, and hasn't had the confidence to ask them about themselves.

I enquire about this lack of confidence holding her back. Her imposter syndrome is still very much present. She feels they got 'the short straw' in having her operate on their dog. She is frightened to let her guard down in front of them in case she gets found out.

For a while we try to imagine what it must be like to be that dog's owners. Ann notes that they were nice to her and didn't question her ability at any stage. She has already said they were polite and compliant.

I ask how she would feel if *her* dog had a large laceration and needed surgery and aftercare. She would be devastated, terrified, sleepless, self-blaming, yearning to turn the clock back.

Sometimes it helps to defuse the hold our emotions are having on us if we give our brains a breather and ask someone else how their day is going, or a bit about themselves, or even the consulting room chat about where someone got their dog from or how their other pets are.

It's also a kind thing to do. Being a pet owner at the vets is usually just as stressful, if not more stressful, than being the vet or the nurse.

Empathy with Owners

We pause to sit with this for a moment.

I ask her how it feels, and Ann says she suddenly feels like there will be a life after being a new grad. She will be beyond a new grad and there is hope on the horizon she will become one of the experienced surgeons.

I ask her about how the wound is at the 10-day mark. Ann stops and looks to the floor. She says 'It's fine but I'm not sure why'.

I ask her if she can probe a little deeper and ask herself why the wound is okay.

Ann feels it is nothing to do with her or her technique. That it's pure chance the wound is okay.

After a pause, I repeat back to her: 'Pure chance?'.

Ann says that she knows her technique was by the book and evidence based. She describes her pre- and post-op care and her surgical technique to me.

She looks for affirmation. I look back and challenge her to challenge her own belief that this is 'pure chance' rather than give her the affirmation she is asking for.

Imposter Syndrome

I ask Ann to close her eyes and we do a breath meditation together, focusing on only the breath for nearly half an hour even though she was to tell me when she was ready to stop. She is becoming experienced at this now.

When she opens her eyes, I ask her to think as clinically as possible and tell me why this wound is 'okay'.

She explains that she followed an evidence-based protocol of pre-op care, surgical technique under supervision and postoperative care. The owners had been compliant because of her good communication. The wound is 'healed'. Actually, it's healed beautifully rather than being just 'okay'.

I challenge Ann. Is the wound healed because of you or in spite of you?

Ann does her own affirmation and says to me that the wound is healed because of everything she did.

We both smile and then she tells me she *was* going to leave the skin sutures in for another week just in case, but that now she will call the owners and take them out at 12 days instead.

I wonder if she can take time in that consult room to get to know the dog and owners a little, to admire her work and to explain to the owners why what she did worked?

Summary

Ann was suffering from anxiety, fear of failure and imposter syndrome when we first met.

Using logic, mindful meditation, MBSR and CBT, she learnt how to stop, pause and clear her mind in order to think rationally about cases.

She learnt how to accept anxiety and all its physical and mental manifestations instead of trying to avoid it and being fearful of anxiety.

At work, she has developed healthy habits of being able to ask for assistance and to discuss cases on a daily basis with all the team.

Using CBT, Ann is able to recognise imposter syndrome in herself and to forgive herself for feeling it. By recognising it and being aware that it will probably happen again, Ann has learnt the skills needed to get affirmation from herself.

Using breathwork, Ann is sleeping better now. She focuses on her breath as soon as she gets to bed. She has better sleep hygiene, leaves the phone down and on silent for an hour before bed and actively chooses to leave work out of her head as soon as she closes her eyes.

Ben (An Experienced Vet)

- First session
- Second session
- Third session
- Summary

Ben is an experienced vet who qualified 15 years ago. He contacted me saying that while he is very comfortable and confident in his clinical work, he feels he has compassion fatigue and doesn't know why or what to do about it.

First Session

When he arrives, I see that Ben is about the same age as me. He says he's happy about that as I may be able to relate to him better than a young therapist or someone outside the profession.

He looks around the room a bit uncomfortably as I go through the explanation that everything said between us is completely confidential.

Then he says, 'I have no idea why I'm here'. He says he doesn't believe in mindfulness, that it's a fad and he's probably just getting a bit bored with his job as opposed to having compassion fatigue.

He says that life is good overall. He goes to the theatre a lot, he has an active social life, all is good at home and he loves to run.

I ask him why he is here and he answers that his practice manager told him to come. We both laugh and can see we would get on as he starts to relax into the sofa and makes friends with my cat.

I explain to him that someone doesn't have to have something 'wrong' with them to have therapy. It can be part of a self-care regime like a workout or a haircut.

Positive psychology is about taking someone from okay to good or from good to great or from great to fantastic.

I ask Ben about his feelings of compassion fatigue and why he had used that term in his email. Ben says that he just doesn't feel any empathy or connection with the clients like he used to do.

Mental Wellbeing and Positive Psychology for Veterinary Professionals: A Pre-emptive, Proactive and Solution-based Approach, First Edition. Laura Woodward.
© 2024 John Wiley & Sons Ltd. Published 2024 by John Wiley & Sons Ltd.

He's doing a good job clinically and his cases benefit from his experience. He helps the younger members of staff and he's always pleasant to people at work, but that he's just going through the motions. It's like he's on auto-pilot.

I ask him if he can remember when he last felt compassion for a client or made a connection with them. He looks to the ceiling for a very long time as if the answer will be there. Then he says it would have been just before the pandemic hit in 2020.

We pause.

I ask Ben to take a few breaths, and to try to clear his head and remember what it felt like to have those connections with an owner and to tell me what he felt.

He chooses to keep his eyes closed and clearly has difficulty remembering emotions from two years previously.

He says he remembers being an animated, respected senior consulting vet. His consult slots were always fully booked and clients would happily wait a few days to see him. He knew their stories, their kids' stories and how he related to them because he has teenage kids like some of them, and he's a dog and cat owner like all of them. He would take a full history, do a good clinical exam and make most diagnoses or diagnostic plans while chatting.

I ask him if he can remember how that felt. He answers, 'It felt normal, good normal'.

I ask him to take a few breaths and get that memory to the front of his mind so he can remember it more easily next time we need it. I think he would have happily kept his eyes closed with that pleasant view for hours had I not asked him to open them again.

I ask Ben to describe how he feels now during a regular consult. He sees what's coming in and knows he can get it done easily and out the door rapidly ready for the next one. He often feels impatience with the owners for not being able to give a full history and answer his questions clearly.

Sometimes he feels angry with the owner if they have left their pet a few days before seeking a consultation.

I ask him about body language and eye contact. Ben feels he doesn't want to connect with the clients any more, he avoids eye contact and asks them only about their pet.

I ask him to compare that to his memory of pre-Covid consultations. He says 'It's like chalk and cheese'. I suggest that maybe it's that chasm between chalk and cheese, between how he was then and how he is now, that has brought him here. He agrees.

I ask him how things were at work during the pandemic. He says he found it unbearable. Although the team at work became very tight-knit and cohesive during the lockdowns, that team was split into two, as were many others, to avoid the entire team becoming infected at once.

He was in a different team from the head nurse who is his friend and they mutually support one another.

Everyone was forging forwards with a 'can do' attitude but he feels he was clinically inept for an entire year and a half. Ben says that 'car park consulting', where he struggled to get a history through a mask, visor and car window, made him feel like he was constantly guessing a diagnosis. He handed out antibiotics like they were going out of fashion.

I ask him if he was doing a good job as a vet during that time and he looks towards the floor. Then he starts to cry.

Ben is surprised at his reaction and his crying. As a counsellor, we always have tissues. Crying in the therapy room means that something is happening.

He says he was a rubbish vet doing a rubbish job during that year and half.

Moral Injury and PTSD

I ask him how he feels about having done a rubbish job for that long. He says he feels ashamed, traumatised and that the way he practised was 'unforgivable'.

I ask how often he has cast his memory back to those days of car park consults. He says he has chosen not to think about it because it's too panful.

I agree that Ben has a degree of compassion fatigue most likely brought on through the moral injury caused by consultations where he couldn't even examine the patient or get a proper history. He has chosen to push this time out of his mind permanently for understandable reasons and I feel for him. We all know what that time felt like. Moral injury is so painful and one of the many reasons why experienced clinicians, including medics, dentists, vets and vet nurses, lie awake at night and leave the professions.

Feeling this intense shame and pain and never saying a word to anyone, not even his friends, choosing instead to power on through, didn't seem to be helping. Because here he was full of pain, unable to glean any joy from his job and unable to communicate with the clients with whom he had connected so easily in the past.

I explain to Ben that mindfulness isn't all about sitting cross-legged on the cushion for an hour. That it isn't magic or wizardry. Mindful meditation can be anything we want it to be. It's basically using your mind to help your mind.

There are many options for us to use in therapy. I suggest using imagery to face this painful experience, to let this monster of pain out of the box and look at it.

We know that with trauma, if we shut it in the box, it will come back time and time again to haunt us. Buddhist psychotherapy is very much about seeing how you are now in this moment, exploring the present you. However, therapy isn't possible without having our backstory out in the open in the counselling room.

I use the analogy of getting a good clinical history in order to be able to sort the condition out, which resonates with Ben, and he agrees to take part in a small mini-meditation just to see what it entails.

I ask Ben to close his eyes and we do a two-minute breath meditation together, just spending two minutes focusing on the breath. When we finish, he opens his eyes and says he really enjoyed having that two-minute 'breather for the mind', like two minutes off the hamster wheel of life.

I ask him if we could do a little more and he is interested now. He closes his eyes and we do a body scan meditation to clear the mind.

Then I ask him to take a look back to the pandemic lockdown time and see a vet in the car park talking to a pet owner in a car. He describes the vet in a gown with a mask and a visor in the rain holding a clipboard and his voice starts to wobble.

I ask him to keep breathing even though it hurts.

We stay like this for some time.

Then I ask Ben if that vet is doing a good job or a rubbish job and he says rubbish.

I ask, if that vet is him from two years ago, is there any way he can find it within himself to forgive that vet for doing a rubbish job, considering everything going on at the time and the inability to even examine the dog in the back of the car?

It's hard to forgive our former selves. If we have spent most of our lives being self-critical or having very high standards, as we typically do in our professions, we hold ourselves to account for every tiny thing we get wrong be it the overuse of antibiotics, an unburied suture, a blown vein or anything else.

If we have done something very wrong, bad or illegal, it's even harder to forgive ourselves. However, it makes it a bit easier to forgive if we try talking to our former selves as though we're talking to another person.

I see that Ben is trying to forgive that poor vet in the rain.

I ask him to open his eyes.

We sit in silence for a bit.

Ben doesn't need to keep going back to that painful memory. He knows it's there now. He has, however, let it out of the box and accepted that it still hurts like hell. However, he has faced it, looked at it and isn't going to try to pretend to himself any more that he is unaffected by it. Because he is deeply affected by moral injury from that time.

Homework

I ask Ben to do one simple task this week. At regular intervals, whenever he thinks of it, he can take a deep breath in and, as he exhales, say to himself in his head the words 'I forgive you', to his former car park consulting self.

Second Session

Ben returns a week later. I ask how he's getting on with his homework. He's finding it simple and likes how he can pepper it throughout his day. He'd like to explore these 'mind games' a bit more. We laugh and agree to call it mind games for now.

I ask him if anything has changed since our first session. Ben says he has opened up to his friend in the practice about the moral injury he suffered during the pandemic and that he feels he has compassion fatigue as a result.

I ask how they reacted and he says they were so supportive and delighted that he had explained a little of what he was feeling to them.

We decide to explore his compassion fatigue a bit more. I ask him to explain how he feels when a client walks into the consult room with their beloved pet. He says he feels himself shut off emotionally and physically from them as they enter.

He can now take a full history like he used to and he can examine the animal excellently, determine a course of action and is happy with his skills again. However, he knows that the client wants more. They want and need a connection he can't give them.

He had thought he'd done a good job of getting over the pandemic but that I had 'opened a can of worms'.

Ben can't tell me why he's putting up the barriers between him and the clients. I suggest it could be because he's scared of letting them down by being rubbish at hs job again.

He pauses for a while and then nods.

Is it safer to never get attached to the owner and the animal? Grief was everywhere during the two years when he was traumatised. Is he associating car park consulting and being rubbish at his job with enormous grief?

Ben nods.

'I can't get emotionally involved with owners in case I return to being rubbish at my job again.'

We do some breathing exercises during which I ask Ben to be present with the pain and grief he is holding. I feel that he has some PTSD associated with the pandemic for multiple reasons.

Then, I turn away from the 'mind games' and to CBT. the barriers are there because he is worried about being rubbish at his job again. And yet, if he knows that he is good clinically and very experienced, is being rubbish at his job again unlikely to happen? Or likely?

Ben says it's unlikely.

I ask him if there are other reasons he won't be in that situation in the rain again. He said that everyone has agreed he wouldn't ever be asked to consult in the car park again.

I challenge him and ask him if he is prepared to take down the barriers between him and the clients again even though it might make him feel vulnerable.

He is open to this but doesn't know how. Rather than me telling him how, a solution or an action is more likely to be valid if Ben comes to it by himself. So I challenge him to come up with some sentence starters, small talk and questions that clients generally are happy to answer.

Ben produces the following suggestions.

- Where did you get his name from?
- Is he your first dog?

- Where do you walk him?
- What toys does your cat like playing with?
- Where do your kids go to school?

Homework

We agree that using these will be his homework for the week. That it may feel a bit rehearsed and insincere but that he will see how it goes.

He is to continue taking one deep breath at regular intervals and forgiving his former self. He even chooses to do 10 minutes of meditation each morning focusing on the breath.

Third Session

Ben is positively bursting with enthusiasm this morning. He is so eager to share his progress and it is wonderful to listen to him and to share in his successes.

He is getting into 'this mindfulness thing' with 10 minutes each morning just holding his coffee and breathing. It is wizardry, he says.

He has changed the words he says in his head to 'It's over and you're forgiven' which makes me feel he is digesting that painful time and putting it into his backstory rather than ignoring it and omitting it from his story all together.

He says he tried a few of the small-talk questions with both new and old clients and finds it has awakened something in him which he had forgotten ever existed. The conversations have started to flow, and he finds he isn't having to make much effort at all. More like the old him again and that it felt amazing.

This last session is short. Ben feels that he is set on a good path now and has much work to do. However, he now feels he can look back at the past and be proud that he had acknowledged at least some of the reasons he was experiencing moral injury and compassion fatigue, and that he can completely absolve himself of being responsible for substandard care during that time.

Summary

Many people have trauma. In fact, everyone has something panful in their past. Only some of us suffer with PTSD. Moral injury is something from which many clinicians never recover. It can become part of our make-up.

Ben needed to forgive himself for something which was not his fault. Sometimes we need to forgive ourselves for something which *is* our fault using the same techniques.

Ben's fear of history repeating itself, with real fear which was shockingly painful, was holding him back and he was possibly in danger of more moral injury or burnout in the future had he continued on that path.

We used CBT to challenge these fears in order that his thoughts would not control his emotions and therefore his actions.

Ben might never recover from the moral injury he suffered because of the pandemic. He may need to incorporate that into his make-up, and the horrors of car park consulting into his backstory.

The hope is that he will be able to practise to a very high standard now and in the future, with compassion and enthusiasm. Also, now that he has experienced mindfulness to a small degree, he says he is keen to explore it further and see how it can benefit him.

Darren (A Specialist Vet)

- First session
- Second session
- Summary

Darren contacted me several times before I met him. He would ask for help, I would reply with empathy and my availability, then I'd hear nothing for six months.

He's a specialist orthopaedic surgeon. When he had a crisis, he would contact me. Then he would put that crisis in a box and move on.

Therapy is never a quick fix to an urgent problem after which we go back to living happily ever after. A crisis has become a crisis because we don't yet have the tools to navigate the inevitable hurdles we are facing.

Even 25 years into the job, Darren was still in denial about his ability to fail. Anything less than success at work would cause him to spiral into a dark place where he could not cope and those around him suffered unbeknown to him.

When Darren spiralled, he would become as egocentric as someone with depression. He simply could not see the havoc he wreaked around him. So the impetus for getting help and the acceptance that he needed help weren't there. He could only see his own suffering. If the pain was slightly eased by two days after a crisis, he felt he was okay.

The third time he contacted me out of the blue asking for an urgent appointment, I challenged him. Either he needed to see what therapy is all about, with me or with another therapist, or he needed to bear this load by himself. He had to make a choice. We met the following week.

First Session

He sat nervously and looked like he would make a bolt for the door any minute.

I explained, as is mandatory, that everything said between us is confidential and even the fact that I have seen him in my counselling rooms is confidential.

Mental Wellbeing and Positive Psychology for Veterinary Professionals: A Pre-emptive, Proactive and Solution-based Approach, First Edition. Laura Woodward.
© 2024 John Wiley & Sons Ltd. Published 2024 by John Wiley & Sons Ltd.

He quizzed me on this and needed reassurance. Darren didn't tell anyone he was having difficulties. Even his wife didn't know he was having crises, he said.

I asked him why he hadn't told anyone or let anyone know. He looked at me as though I had asked the most ridiculous question on earth. In fairness, it's quite a difficult starter question.

I told him I could sense he was in a hurry to get therapy over and done with, like drive-thru therapy, and he laughed and relaxed a little.

Darren had never let anyone know he had any problems for as long as he could remember. He tried to remember university, then secondary school and even primary school and just could not remember the last time he had admitted he was unable to succeed.

He is a very competent skier. Even when learning that, he said, he had private lessons in secret before he allowed anyone to see him ski.

I asked him to sit with that secret for a minute. Then I asked him to take some time to see if he could figure out why he had taken those lessons in secret. After a long pause, Darren said he cares a lot about what people think of him. He never dances in case he looks awkward, he tends to his social media image daily, and he said he craves online 'likes'.

At work, he presumes everyone's judging him. He said 'You're only ever as good as your last TPLO (tibial plateau levelling osteotomy)'.

I understand that sentiment. The praise we get for a challenging fracture repair is only one broken bone away from shame and embarrassment. And, as the surgeon, only we truly know that feeling.

'How was your last TPLO?' I asked. 'Good' he replied.

'And the one before that?' 'Also good.'

'When did you last have a surgery which went badly?'

Darren was clearly struggling with my being a vet. And yet he had come to me for therapy, on purpose, for this very reason.

About four weeks previously, Darren had had a fracture failure. He had repaired a straightforward femoral fracture with locking plate and screws. The plate had broken. He had blamed the owner. He had revised it with double plating 'in anger' as he described it. Now the dog had an osteomyelitis with discharging tracts.

He knew how to manage this case. As a specialist, he had seen dozens of cases like this although usually the osteomyelitis or implant failures were someone else's repairs being referred in.

I asked him, if it wasn't the management of this case which was causing him such distress, what were the emotions he felt which had the enormous effect of getting him here?

He took some time to answer and then said he wasn't used to anything but perfection from himself. This wasn't the first case to go wrong for him this year and he felt he was losing his skill set. He also felt that his eyesight wasn't as good as it had been when he was younger and no amount of different contact lenses, surgical lights or loupes could make his vision as good as before.

I asked him about wearing glasses. He said he avoids this as much as possible and never wears glasses at work for fear people will think he's getting old and judge him for it.

So Darren was fearful of ageing and of how people would judge him for this. He was fearful of the effects of ageing and angry that he couldn't stay at the top of his game for ever.

He was angry and ashamed that he was down-skilling possibly due to his eyesight changing, and blaming poor outcomes on owners, faulty autoclaves, etc.

And he had no coping skills for any of these difficulties, because he had never needed coping skills like this before. He had never learned them as a child, never been taught them by his parents, and never saw the need for these 'hippy soft skills'.

Wanting to lighten the mood for a bit, I asked him what he did with his free time. He did very little. He didn't enjoy holidays as they never lived up to his expectations. He didn't have children. Physical fitness and sport were things he'd hated as a schoolchild and he wasn't likely to take up anything like that, apart from the skiing, since he was freed from the school PE curriculum. He'd never pursued any creative hobbies because they didn't seem useful on his path.

When he read, it was either self-help books or books about business management and orthopaedics.

I asked a challenging question: what did he see himself doing when he retired? He sighed. Clearly, this was not what he had come here to discuss. The problem was acute. Talking about retirement was irrelevant.

I knew that. The point of asking this question was to see if he believed that there would be an endpoint to his career. He had purposefully never allowed himself to consider this endpoint. It was too frightening. There was a cliff face at the end of his career and a deep, dark, end-of-the-earth type fall over the edge. It was easier to not consider this.

I asked Darren if he would be okay to sit with these uncomfortable feelings for a while and he agreed.

Visualising retirement and this cliff face and darkness beyond, I asked if he could allow himself to believe that this will happen. It's not a question of if but when. It is uncomfortable now and it will probably be terrifying then, but facing it pre-emptively would mean it's less likely to end in a massive crisis.

Sometimes, when we have uncomfortable emotions like these, it can help to take a sideways glance at them, knowing and accepting that they exist and that the cause of them exists.

We are aware of them in our peripheral vision. We don't have to like them but not being shocked by them when those causes are realised will save us from the impending doom we presume they will bring.

After this exercise, I asked Darren how he felt.

He felt 'surprisingly relieved'.

'In what way?'

Darren had put the thought of his career drawing to a close in a box of avoidable nightmares for so long, he felt relieved that he could actually look at these frightening thoughts and for it not to have any dire consequences. It was, after all, only looking. It was probably 5–15 years away.

I asked Darren if he would come back and commit to seeing what we could do together if we really dug into these difficulties. Luckily, he was enthused, and a bit interested in therapy and psychology by now.

Homework

For the first week, I asked him to practise a basic body scan meditation each morning for 10 minutes just to get used to a new soft skill. I talked him through this and we did it together in the first session.

At the end of this 10 minutes, I wanted him to take a few sideways glances at the distant future and then bring his attention back to the present, just to acknowledge that there would be changes coming.

I also gave him a copy of Part One, Chapter 4 on the nature of impermanence to see what he thought, especially in relation to his eyesight, potential down-skilling and beyond.

Second Session

I was a bit sceptical whether Darren would return the next week, but he was on time and eager to get going.

I asked him how his week and the exercises I gave him had gone. He found it quite easy to do the exercises, the chapter had been interesting and his week had been uneventful.

I asked him what uneventful meant to him. I know what it means to me. Nothing had gone wrong. So we probably had a similar idea of what uneventful means at work.

However, the difference between us was that I would rejoice with 'uneventful' because nothing happening is fantastic considering all the things which can go wrong at work.

We had a bit of a fun back-and-forth where Darren said 'nothing going wrong' is his role as a specialist. I challenged this and said that his cases will be harder than mine as I'm not a specialist. So surely 'nothing going wrong' for him was even more worthy of celebration. He then said that he couldn't accept something going wrong.

I asked him what this non-acceptance felt like. It would make him quiet and yet he wanted to scream at the same time. He would be monosyllabic at best, even at home, if he had an ongoing complication, until it was fixed.

I asked if he ever leant on his colleagues emotionally when he had an ongoing difficult case. He didn't. He had never leant on anyone, not his wife, his family nor his colleagues. He had been an A* student since he could talk (he said) and that was his only quality.

'Your only quality?'

Darren is a vet at the top of his game. He said it's the only game he can play and that being at the top is the only place he's ever been. He had gone from graduating, to residency to lectureship to specialist referral centre.

His big secret is that only he knows how narrow his skill set actually is. He said he is incapable of doing anything else.

I asked him why he felt his colleagues would judge him harshly when he had a complication or a difficult case, rather than supporting him.

He wasn't sure.

I asked him what emotions *he* would feel if his colleague had a plate break or another fracture failure. His answer, he later said, shocked him as he said it. He would feel a bit smug, also grateful it wasn't his case, and 'possibly, no probably' judge them harshly out loud and to others.

I asked Darren how he feels and acts when he is referred a case for revision. He said similar to this.

I was so grateful for his honesty. The client–therapist relationship relies heavily on honesty on both sides and mutual positive regard.

I put it to him that it could be his fear of others judging him harshly and out loud, as he does, that makes him terrified of being imperfect. Darren agreed that he was indeed fearful of being treated the way he treats others.

And yet, his colleagues weren't like him. They were supportive, open, honest and imperfect and a great deal more content at work than he was.

I asked him why he judges others out loud.

'Habit' he replied. He said that he had been doing it for as long as he could remember.

We sat in silence for a bit.

'I suppose it makes me look better when I make others look worse.'

I asked him if it made him *feel* better as well as his perception that it made him look better.

He said that was a harsh realisation. No, it probably made him feel worse, and made him even more secretive about his imperfections, and more on the periphery of the team who were generally mutually supportive.

I asked him, if he's been doing this for as long as he can remember, could he guess when it started? As a child, he replied.

I looked at him inquisitively. He realised he was being child-like, and not in the wonderful, awe-struck way we talked about earlier but rather in an immature way while living in a very adult mature professional environment. This mismatch was unlikely to be helpful.

Homework

It may seem easy but after 25 years of behaving a certain way, it takes courage and focus to change.

I asked Darren to continue his morning body scan practice and to extend it to 20 minutes. I also asked him to read the chapter on Empathy and to see if he could visualise where the different types of empathy might feature in his life at work and at home.

Finally, he was to add in an exercise at work where he would learn to stop, pause and think about the impact of his words before he said them;

for example, if he was angry with himself, he would stop, breathe, choose his reaction, proceed.

If seeing a second opinion case he feels has been mismanaged – stop, breathe, consider the impact of his words on the owners, the referring practice, his success (and whether his words really do affect his success) before speaking.

And so on.

Third Session

Darren reported feeling brighter this week. He wasn't really sure why.

He'd had a luxation of a total hip replacement he'd done. He'd reacted differently to it from how he would have reacted before.

I asked in what way.

He said he'd been practising the stopping, pausing and choosing his outward and inward reactions carefully with the simple run-of-the-mill cases. However, when this luxation happened, that exercise went out the window because he was so embarrassed and ashamed.

The change was that although the emotions of shame and embarrassment were present, there was no anger, he didn't feel like blaming the owners and he didn't seem to want to let the expletives rip.

I put it to Darren that maybe the exercises he had been doing when it was easy were kicking into action when he needed them the most, and that his efforts were indeed paying off.

He was unused to these soft skills and found it difficult to see when he was succeeding at them. There's no doubt that success with mindfulness is difficult to measure without a functional MRI.

Regarding the luxation, he didn't need to do a complete revision and he managed it appropriately. The dog was doing fine now.

I asked what he'd thought about the lengthy piece on Empathy. He'd found it interesting. Then he asked me if I thought he was a narcissist.

In TV sitcoms, therapists often answer a question with another question. That can be so useful. But Darren had been sitting on this question for a week and needed affirmation.

Yes, he is a fantastic surgeon, but with little or no confidence. Narcissists typically lack emotional empathy although they may have shedloads of cognitive empathy.

I did feel that Darren was lacking in emotional empathy but I didn't think he was narcissistic. It's not pathognomonic.

It's possible that he was not taught emotional empathy by example when he was growing up.

Often, if you're secretly frightened while walking in your own shoes, it's even more terrifying to step into someone else's. Darren could see that he has high levels of cognitive empathy with good communication skills. However, he used those skills only when he wanted and when it wouldn't make him feel even more vulnerable to judgement by others.

When it came to emotional empathy, it was difficult to understand what it meant or felt like. We chatted about my understanding of emotional empathy being that you feel an internal, visceral reaction when someone near you shows emotion or talks about their emotions. That feeling might be joy because of someone else's joy. Or it might be heart ache when someone you care about or even a stranger on the news is in turmoil.

It's important to differentiate between what emotions are ours and ours alone and what emotions are those of others to which we relate.

Darren had felt nothing when his wife's mother died. Literally nothing, he said. He had reacted to the news by organising work around the funeral arrangements, telling his wife that her mum's death was inevitable and trying to relate but not 'getting it'. In fact, he said, he had never felt the grief his parents or any other bereaved people had felt, and that he had felt devoid of emotion when they were that upset.

That was what had made him ask me if I was a narcissist.

I wondered if he could 'dip his toe in' and start to explore this a little more very gradually, in small increments, just to see how it felt and to observe others' reactions which he feared so much.

To start with, maybe he could check himself when others were speaking and really lean into what they were saying and also what they weren't saying. Also, actively listening by pausing instead of feeling that need to respond reflexively.

This would be difficult, he said.

The pace and size of these increments are completely under his control. However, he's spent his entire life until now shielding himself from other people's emotions as well as his own for fear it might make him vulnerable.

I asked him what it would feel like to be vulnerable emotionally.

He answered 'A bit like I do now because you're challenging me'.

Could he accept those feelings of vulnerability? Maybe frame them as a new awakening and exciting time although very uncomfortable.

He was willing to try.

We did a short exercise together using self-awareness skills. Darren imagined himself opening up to a loved one, describing his insecurity about something he chose. This first time it was about his eyesight failing.

He observed and named the physical sensations of anxiety and disgust, and his emotional response of terror and desperation for positive affirmation. I asked him to breathe and to stay with those emotions for as long as he could.

Then we took a few breaths together and he opened his eyes.

Homework

I asked Darren to see if he could do this exercise a few times at home, visualising different people and opening up about other difficulties. Then to put it into practice at work and at home.

I also asked him to read the piece about resilience (Part six, Chapter six), and in particular its relationship with mindfulness. Resilience means different things to different people. In his case, I believed Darren's mindfulness practice, which had been going on for two weeks straight by now, was helping with his resilience when it came to surgical complications.

He agreed.

So, if he was becoming stronger at coping with adversity in the workplace, my hope was that he would become stronger and feel less vulnerable and frightened of the prospect of his eyesight fading further and the possibility he might start to down-skill in the coming years.

Summary

Darren had spent the vast majority of his life achieving what appeared to be the ideal: fantastic grades, career escalation to the pinnacle, a loving wife.

He had many vulnerabilities and difficulties which were increasing in number as he became older and which he kept to himself. He also kept the ensuing emotional difficulties to himself.

His habit of judging others in order to make himself look better was also detrimental to his mental wellbeing.

It had taken some time for him to trust another person with this enormous mental load. His strength of character in opening up cannot be overestimated.

He was willing to try new techniques after a lifetime of resisting change and this courage was starting to pay off.

Using mindfulness and meditation along with reading materials and his own online research, he was starting to come to terms with the nature of impermanence and the inevitable physical changes middle age brings.

His resilience in the face of difficulties was increasing due to his mindfulness practice and he could see the evidence base for this.

When feeling stronger about facing the present and near future, he will proceed to look at the distant future with more than just a sideways glance.

He was dipping his toe into opening up to vulnerability and the anxiety it can bring using role play and imagery and then applying it to real life at home and at work.

He wanted to increase his emotional empathy and now knows how to. He wants to become a less judgemental team member at work and be less on the periphery.

He also wants to be able to glean support from his colleagues when surgical complications happen.

He wants to have more emotional empathy and a greater connection with his wife and he will work on this.

Darren had many more sessions after these and continued to up-skill emotionally after a great many years of suffering in silence.

Claire (Head Nurse)

- First session
- Second session
- Summary

Claire contacted me a short time after being promoted to the role of head nurse because she felt 'stressed and out of her depth'.

Claire had started her job as a veterinary receptionist shortly after her GCSEs. It was meant to be an interim job while she decided what to do next. She was thinking of joining a performing arts college but her parents wanted 'more' for her and were not willing to fund her place.

She wanted to save money for college. Meanwhile she was living with her girlfriend to avoid 'aggro' from her parents.

At the practice, Claire was liked by the team, she enjoyed meeting the clients and was interested in her work. She felt she was making friends who accepted and valued her. She would read the clinical notes and histories and felt included in the care of the patients.

She had been in this post for several years when she became a bit bored.

The college of performing arts was increasing its fees annually, COVID had increased the demand for places there after two years with a decreased number of overseas students, and Claire had felt she wanted to be proactive about her future.

She enrolled as a PCA/ACA with a view to training as a nurse when a student place became available at her practice.

The team had been very supportive and enthusiastic about Claire joining the clinical side. A place became available and she was the obvious choice to fill this slot.

She worked hard at work and at college, her relationship with her girlfriend and her parents was solid, and she qualified after two years. This brought a pay rise, a great feeling of achievement and Claire had felt that she was in a better place to pursue both this career and a career in the performing arts once she became sufficiently established that she could work part time as a nurse.

However, when the role of head nurse became available, Claire had felt she ought to apply because it was a good promotion, her parents and

Mental Wellbeing and Positive Psychology for Veterinary Professionals: A Pre-emptive, Proactive and Solution-based Approach, First Edition. Laura Woodward.
© 2024 John Wiley & Sons Ltd. Published 2024 by John Wiley & Sons Ltd.

girlfriend had encouraged her to apply and the team were very keen for her to fill the role. It was advertised externally as well. Claire was undecided about it but 'before she realised it' she was head nurse.

The stress started pretty much 'from the word go' she said. She had received a significant pay rise and had a lot of new tasks in addition to those she already had as a newly qualified nurse.

She felt out of her depth with the number of new jobs she had to do and the perceived level of knowledge others felt she had, which she knew she didn't.

She was being asked clinical questions which she couldn't answer due to her lack of experience, and she felt stressed and overwhelmed.

First Session

I had never met Claire before, but I could see that she looked tired and stressed as soon as we met.

She told me her story at speed and with the efficiency that I imagine made her attractive to the workplace and the team.

I asked her if it was okay for us to draw a timeline on a large sheet of poster paper so it might be easier to visualise. Sometimes artistic people like to work with visuals. She was a very visual person she said so that would work.

So, we plotted out her journey from GCSEs to now along a line and it was obvious how fast her career had taken off. She knew why this was and she was proud of her achievements, but pride wasn't helping her to deal with the accompanying stress and feelings of being overwhelmed.

Seeing as how Claire was a visual person, I asked her if she would be keen on doing an exercise with imagery and she was.

I taught her how to clear her mind using a simple breath meditation and I could sense she was relaxed.

I asked her to imagine a conveyor belt in front of her. All the 'items' would wait in a pile on the left. Then, one by one, they would hop onto the conveyor belt, appear in her line of vision like on a TV screen, there would be a pause while she looked at the item, then it would pass along and the next item would appear.

The pile of 'items' was a mixture of tasks and concerns.

I talked her through this exercise, reminding her occasionally that she was looking at each item non-judgementally, just observing it and then allowing it to pass.

She continued to do this for several minutes. I kept gently reminding her to keep going.

After about 15 minutes, I asked Claire to open her eyes and tell me how she'd got on. She was surprised that she'd run out of items after about half the time. Each time I reminded her to keep going, she'd search for another task but had already accounted for all of them.

This was the object of the exercise, I said: first of all, to see that the list is finite. We often feel so overwhelmed by our list that we just start with what we can see and plough on through at speed in the hope we get it all done.

Her list was finite, but it was also too long for anyone, even one as efficient as Claire, to deal with.

I asked her how she felt.

She liked the breath meditation as a break from the turmoil of her life and she was pleased that the list was in fact finite. But, she added, she would never be able to get through that list.

That, I felt, was a revelation and something which Claire had never realised before. She hadn't had enough time to see that she didn't have enough time to do everything.

I wondered how it had become so. She thought for a while and said that with the promotion and increase in pay came an increase in duties.

That's true in most jobs, I suppose. However, promotions don't increase the number of hours in each day and Claire was doing many hours of overtime and still not getting all her nursing jobs completed along with her head nurse jobs. She was taking work home (rotas, etc.) and there was no let-up in the list.

I wondered if she had talked this over with her line manager. Claire said she didn't have one as such, it was probably the head vet.

She hadn't been given a job description and she hadn't asked for one.

I asked if she would feel comfortable having a conversation with the head vet to see if her role could become more definite and more possible given the number of hours in each day.

Claire didn't want to admit the role was 'beyond her'. She had been a high achiever since entering the practice. She was surrounded by high achievers who cared about her and she felt like she belonged.

She had risen up 'through the ranks' to this position and was proud of this. However, the role took up more hours in the day than even she could manage. Yet, Claire felt unable to advocate for herself.

I asked if we could explore this a bit further.

Lack of assertiveness and being unable to advocate for oneself can become paralysing when in a senior role. It can lead to burnout and to great people leaving their posts if left unaddressed.

I asked Claire whether her lack of assertiveness at home had become the norm for her. Her parents had disapproved of her wanting to go to the college of performing arts and Claire had gone along with their wishes instead of advocating for herself.

She agreed that she doesn't speak up at home for fear of rocking the boat. What would happen if she rocked the boat? Claire sighed and shrugged her shoulders. She wasn't sure.

Could she imagine what would happen? She said probably nothing that awful. Maybe her parents would express their disappointment and not be very encouraging.

Would anything else happen?

She felt that would be it, really. She didn't doubt their love for her and she knew they'd get over their disappointment rather than there being any big falling out.

In that case, I asked, wouldn't it be worth 'rocking the boat' in order to pursue what *she* wanted?

She said she'd never thought it worth the fallout but that now she realised the fallout wasn't actually something worth fearing because it would be mild, maybe she should have advocated for herself.

In any case, that was the past and we're here now.

So what would be the fallout of her speaking with the head vet about her concerns?

Claire smiled – again probably not as bad or intolerable as she had feared but still something she didn't want to do.

I respected her opinion, of course.

Homework

I asked Claire to practise the mindful breathing meditation each morning for 10 minutes before looking at her phone. Then she could do the conveyor belt meditation we'd practised for some reassurance that, although there were still too many tasks, the list was finite.

I also asked her to be creative with a pros and cons list of advocating for herself in the future to her line manager.

Finally, I gave her a copy of Lack of Assertiveness Part three, Chapter seven to read.

Second Session

I asked Claire how she'd got on with the homework tasks. She had found the breath meditation nearly impossible. Thoughts, to-do lists and stresses intruded on her mind every time she'd attempted it. Although she was pushing them out of her mind, it took the full 10 minutes to get into that space where her mind was clear even for a moment.

She'd liked the chapter on assertiveness and loved The Killers' lyrics and music.

The conveyor belt meditation had been helpful in calming her down when she was feeling overwhelmed and short of breath.

I asked her to bring her pros and cons list.

The cons list, she said, was less unbearable than she'd imagined. It consisted more of her uncomfortable emotions and physical feelings than it did of actual life-changing consequences. For example, she would be adding to her stressors by calling that meeting, she would be short of breath before it, lose sleep and feel nauseous.

Even though you've said the consequences are less terrifying than the meeting itself?

Yes.

What about the pros? This was a long list.

She could present her idea of an achievable list of tasks for the head nurse role.

She could show the managers of the practice how to write an accurate job description and in that way be advocating not only for herself but for all the staff.

She would hopefully be able to return to enjoying her job. So she might stay in the role which she knew everyone wanted her to do.

She could learn how to charge for overtime and set up a system whereby everybody could do this as there wasn't one in place at the moment. This was a good management skill. She would be paid for the job she was doing instead of being paid for one role while doing two.

She would be advocating for herself rather than being an onlooker onto her life. This was a life skill that could have a real impact on her life at work, at home, with her girlfriend.

I asked Claire if now that she could compare one list with another, she would be more inclined to advocate for herself with her line manager and she said she definitely would.

She first wanted to make out a clear plan for how she saw her role, her duties and the hours she would need to complete these tasks, ideally without having to do overtime.

Going back to advocating for herself outside work, I asked her how she would use this new skill, bearing in mind that she said she would be able to use it in her life with her long-term girlfriend.

Claire said that she was 'guilty' of not standing up for herself with her girlfriend Mim. As they lived in Mim's flat, Claire felt she was very much the tenant and Mim the landlord.

That was partly why she had a massive lists of tasks at home after work. She would clean, shop and cook much more than Mim. Claire was exhausted and felt that it was a mirror of her work: a never-ending list of things which needed to be done by her.

She was indeed the tenant and Mim the landlord.

I asked if she did this instead of paying rent.

Claire sighed. No, she paid rent as well.

I asked why.

Claire supposed that it's similar to work where she felt her promotion brought with it a long list of extra tasks to be squeezed into the day somehow. Living with Mim, although she paid normal rent, brought with it a list of tasks she did to 'justify her place there'.

Justify what, I asked.

Claire shrugged. She didn't know.

Had Mim asked her to do this? No, it was self-imposed.

We could look at this two different ways. Either here is history repeating itself and Claire is doubly in trouble, or now that she has these newly learned skills of advocating for herelf and writing pros and cons lists, she could tackle this problem in the same way. If she believed that it was a problem, of course.

At the end of that session, Claire left with the intention of using her assertiveness skills to make her home life as high quality as her work life.

Summary

Claire continues to meditate and has set up a meditation hub at her practice with noise-cancelling headphones, meditation apps and incense. She had a whirlwind rise to the position of head nurse without a job description. By learning to advocate for herself, she has made significantly beneficial changes to her home life, work life and to the practice management structure. Advocating for oneself and being assertive can be seen as a kind thing to do for those around us. Because of Claire, the head vet has learnt how to make the roles more structured and has learnt that they need to be more tuned in to the staff who are saying very little. Claire is now job-sharing the role of head nurse and has started at a College of Performing Arts near to the practice.

Part 6

Positive Psychology

My mission in life is not merely to survive, but to thrive; and to do so with some passion, some compassion, some humour, and some style. Surviving is important. Thriving is elegant.

Maya Angelou

Gratitude

- What gratitude isn't
- Grateful for nothing

Gratitude practice is the mindful noticing of whatever we can appreciate. Sometimes it's simply noticing that nothing bad happened that day.

Try this experiment. Try to feel grateful that something good is happening. Now try to feel angry about something at the same time.

It's difficult, isn't it? Too conflicting to be feeling both at the same time?

In this section, Chapter 7 we will talk about two ways of looking at something.

Sometimes we have multiple emotions about different things at the same time. For example you might be delighted with the weather and sad for your bereaved friend simultaneously. Possibly you can do it, but it may be difficult.

> With practice, we can experience feeling uplifting gratitude and feeling sadness or grief simultaneously, the gratitude softening the effect of the sadness.

Try this practice.

Close your eyes and take a few breaths. Feel grateful that you are alive, can breathe, don't have lung disease or even a cold. Really notice the inward and outward movement of the breath. Can you feel grateful for a minute that this is happening 24/7 even when we're unconscious? It's so simple. It took no planning, it costs nothing and breathing requires zero concentration. And therein lies both the problem and the potential.

It requires no concentration. So, it gets no attention.

So why focus on it? It isn't a problem which needs to be solved so why should I give it my valuable attention?

The answer is that the benefits of gratitude are so obvious from the first gratitude practice you do that it would be madness not to try it.

What Gratitude Isn't

Gratitude is *not* positive thinking. It isn't turning that frown upside down or seeing that every cloud has a silver lining.

Mental Wellbeing and Positive Psychology for Veterinary Professionals: A Pre-emptive, Proactive and Solution-based Approach, First Edition. Laura Woodward.
© 2024 John Wiley & Sons Ltd. Published 2024 by John Wiley & Sons Ltd.

It's not a cliché.

Neither is it saying thank you or the giving of gifts, although they are wonderful symbols of gratefulness and very worthwhile.

Gratitude practice is the mindful noticing of whatever we can appreciate.

When Buddhist monks wake up, unlike the rest of us who start doom scrolling even before the first coffee's started, they feel gratitude for the fact that they have woken up. They take a breath and feel grateful for it, they feel the ground beneath their feet, see the light if the sun has risen and start their day happier and healthier as a result.

> *Instead of having a fault-finding mind, develop the beautiful attitude of gratitude.*
>
> Ajahn Brahm

It's not rocket science. We can all do it.

Tomorrow, when your alarm goes off, try taking the first minute out of your day to switch your mindset from 'Ugh, not already' to 'I'm grateful for...' (you decide).

Yes, it may sound unrealistic and hippy. I'm not suggesting you glibly repeat any words while thinking about what you need to wear today. Of course, you tailor the mantra to yourself to make it more valid. But I'm asking that you try it for just a week. Write it down when you go to bed, three things you're grateful for. Read it when you get up and also add three basics in the morning like being able to breathe, drink clean water, walk, etc.

Notice if it has any effect on your mood.

Have you ever woken up in a bad mood for no obvious reason? The first emotion you feel as you rise is being fed up? It's not a cheerful way to start the day. That's not a judgement, it's just an observation.

What if we could turn that around so that every day, our mantra of gratitude could provide us with at least the chance of having an open, upbeat attitude and start to the day?

Grateful for Nothing

In a light-hearted way, being grateful for nothing is the easiest gratitude practice of all. Gregg Krech asks 'When was the last time you felt grateful because nothing happened? Nobody crashed into your car. The electricity didn't go out. You didn't wake up with a toothache?' (Krech 2017).

'Nothing happened' isn't particularly exciting. It's not as entertaining as a good movie. It's not intellectually challenging, nor is it adorable like a spaniel puppy. But when you expect the worst and nothing happens, it's worthy of celebration. A celebration of the fact that despite all our problems and aches and pains and financial challenges and relationship conflicts, we're alive and we're breathing and at the moment, we're safe. So, take a moment and sit back. And breathe in 'nothing happened'. And breathe out a breath of thanks. Gratitude for just being able to breathe. Now that's really something!

At work, if none of our patients bleed or die, we barely notice it. It's acceptable, satisfactory, as it should be, for goodness sake. But maybe we should take more notice of what went right and what didn't go wrong.

Try this practice.

Close your eyes and picture someone very dear to you. It might be your child, your pet, your partner.

Now try to list a few things you are grateful for on their behalf. Sometimes it's easier to be grateful for the good things that happen to our *loved* ones compared to those that happen to us directly.

For example, I'm grateful every morning that all my cats are alive, well and yelling at me for food. Nothing happened to them during the night.

I'm grateful every day that my children get in from school. Whatever mood they're in, they didn't get knocked down by a bus.

I'm grateful looking out the window that no trees fell down on my garden during the winds last night.

I'm even grateful that our sunflower seeds have sprouted into seedlings without being used as a litter tray.

It may feel like an effort at the start, noticing the teeny tiny good things or 'lack of bad things' all around us. Don't worry. It's not insincere. You can be aware of the grave horrific atrocities in your life and in the world simultaneously while doing gratitude practice.

The point is that we know that gratitude practice makes us feel better, helps us to cope with the tough stuff in life, makes our loved ones feel more at ease around us. So, instead of putting off this new morning habit until we get the 'right moment', we could just do it now.

There's a story about a monk who carried water from a well in two buckets, one of which had holes in it. He did this every day, without repairing the bucket. One day, a passer-by asked him why he continued to carry the leaky bucket. The monk pointed out that the side of the path where he carried the full bucket was barren, but on the other side of the path where the bucket had leaked, beautiful wildflowers had flourished.

He noticed and felt gratitude.

Reference

Krech, G. (2017). *Question Your Life: Naikan Self-Reflection and the Transformation of our Stories*. Monkton, VT: ToDo Institute Books.

Kindness

- Small acts of kindness
- Random acts of kindness

> *We cannot do great things on this earth, only small things with great love.*
>
> Mother Teresa

Whether you think she was deserving of sainthood or possessed by the devil in her later years, the fact remains that Mother Teresa was truly content. She lived to a fantastic age of 87, she felt deeply loved and she had a positive impact on thousands of individuals: things that many of us aspire to.

Contentment, feeling love and affecting people around us in a positive way are totally within our grasp, and one way we can achieve them is through performing so-called random acts of kindness on a daily basis as our new normal.

Small Acts of Kindness

Lending a helping hand to a co-worker who's behind on their consults or ops list, even though this means that you will have to stay late at work.

Make someone a tea without asking if they want one. Whether they drink tea or not, they will feel that you care.

When driving, allowing others out into the line of traffic is not just good driving and keeping the flow of cars going, it can make your journey and your day feel better. And if they thank you, try thanking them for thanking you. Honestly, I've been doing this for years and it feels great. The look of surprise on the other driver's face is comical, but they drive on happier and so do you.

Phoning or visiting someone who has been bereaved a few months after their loss. There are crowds of helpers around when our loved one

Mental Wellbeing and Positive Psychology for Veterinary Professionals: A Pre-emptive, Proactive and Solution-based Approach, First Edition. Laura Woodward.
© 2024 John Wiley & Sons Ltd. Published 2024 by John Wiley & Sons Ltd.

dies and in the few weeks afterwards. Then people get back to their normal routine and yet the bereaved are still in need of that company.

Here's a good one for Londoners. When you squeeze onto the packed tube with someone's armpit resting neatly over your face, try, instead of feeling hatred towards your fellow commuters, making yourself realise that they are actually just like you (stating the obvious). Maybe try to wish them well, happiness and peace. This has to be in your thoughts though and not out loud, of course. But when you scan the carriage and see the bowed heads of people frantically scanning their phones, avoiding eye contact and not enjoying their journey either, and you feel compassion and kindness towards them, it really can make for a more positive commute and a sense of acceptance and calm within.

Kindness is a trait which is often undervalued or seen as being 'soft'. Some more cynical people see others who are driven by kindness as 'enablers' or 'suckers'. This reflects a belief system where success is only achieved through stepping on or ignoring others – a belief system which is rife in the veterinary world.

I have yet to meet a truly content cynic.

Maybe us 'soft suckers' are perpetuating this belief system by *apologising* for being a bit hippy when we advocate random acts of kindness towards fellow malodorous commuters, instead of unapologetically *promoting* this behaviour as a route to true contentment.

In 2006, in a study of Japanese undergraduates, Otake and colleagues found that happy people were kinder than people who were not happy. Which came first? The happiness or the kindness? Or is it a self-perpetuating cycle? (Kerr et al. 2015, Otake et al. 2006). Their study also revealed that one's sense of happiness was increased by the simple act of counting one's acts of kindness. This is something to do at the end of the day just before sleep.

It's like the typical act of 'helping the little old lady to cross the street'. You feel good about yourself, she feels heartfelt gratitude that someone cares and that she had a moment of connection with a kind person today. It's a win–win situation.

Changing our focus and looking around us, we will notice a multitude of opportunities for kindness. Letting someone into the line of traffic and thanking them for thanking you (or at least not hating them for *not* thanking you), allowing someone to get off the tube in front of you, thanking the guy in Costa for making your coffee just how you like it, dropping a thank-you note in to the people downstairs who always accept your Amazon parcels for you. It takes no time or intelligence to suss out these opportunities. It provides a wholesome opportunity for releasing a warm burst of endorphins and the rewards are instant and last for as long as we decide. It's a cheap and healthy high.

Random Acts of Kindness

When you are kind to others, having that awareness heightens the sense of your own good fortune.

Also, random acts of kindness promote empathy and compassion which in turn lead to a sense of interconnectedness with others. Human interconnectedness is vital for good mental wellbeing.

Feeling connected melds us together rather than dividing us. Kindness is potent in strengthening a sense of community and belonging.

Kindness is not random, it is done on purpose.

Sonia Withrow

References

Kerr, S.L., O'Donovan, A., and Pepping, C.A. (2015). Can gratitude and kindness interventions enhance well-being in a clinical sample? *Journal of Happiness Studies* 16: 17–36.

Otake, K., Shimai, S., Tanaka-Matsumi, J. et al. (2006). Happy people become happier through kindness: a counting kindnesses intervention. *Journal of Happiness Studies* 7: 361–375.

Mindful Gift Giving and Receiving

- How to practise mindful gift giving
- Mindful receiving of gifts

The giving and receiving of gifts has the potential to be a wholesome and comforting experience where we show kindness and affection to our loved ones and feel it radiating back from them to us.

Enormous posters and full-page ads on our screens show us just how Christmas, Thanksgiving, Chanukah and Divali 'ought' to look like if we do it right. We should have the perfect mood lighting, a magnificently laid table with a good-looking heterosexual couple and their two joyful children exchanging large gifts with delight, the magnificent spread in the background promising a sumptuous meal with all the trimmings which are never cold, soggy or burnt.

However, the reality is that while we may strive to make our day look just like that, it rarely does.

We can choose to enjoy whatever parts of the festivities go relatively well or we can choose to become stressed about the cooking, the gift buying, the costs of everything. We can feel unmoved by the gifts we receive, especially if they've obviously been re-gifted to us. We can buy just any old thing for someone out of obligation or reciprocation or because it was three for the price of two, or we can take time out of our crazy schedule to choose gifts to give with mindfulness and thought.

Part One, Chapter One shows how we can squeeze mindful living into our day as a vet or nurse, and how we can do mini-meditations because we don't have time to spare for full-blown sitting-on-the-cushion meditations.

I know how taking one breath, inhaling and exhaling may be the only six seconds in the day we can spare to notice the here and now, because I work in an insanely busy practice too.

I understand that, at home, multitasking is cooking food while emailing, while emptying the dishwasher, filling it and hanging up clothes simultaneously during a Facetime call.

Yet now, I'm asking you to spend time you really don't have on gift shopping.

The big family celebration for many people is a stressful day. A day where close relatives are holed up together whether they like it or not. Or it might be a day of painful loneliness, full of yearning for company or wishing that one's family was intact. Or we might be remembering and longing for those who have died.

For others, it might be their favourite day of the year, when kids are full of sugar and excitement, the prosecco is flowing and someone else is cooking.

We might be devastated or delighted or nonplussed that we're working.

Most people feel their day is something in between, or a mixture of all of the above.

When it comes to giving gifts, we can get so much pleasure and joy from seeing the look on someone's face when they see what we've given them, and they are genuinely delighted with it. We glean joy from seeing the happiness of those we love.

> It's not how much we give, but how much care we put into giving that matters.

How to Practise Mindful Gift Giving

When starting to choose the gift, think of the person with loving kindness when deciding what you want to give to them Part Two, Chapter One. Think about your relationship with them and the good feelings which come with that. Consider what would bring them joy. It's not always the most expensive or flashy item.

My mum would always reply with the same answer when we asked her what she'd like for her birthday. She'd ask for something we had made ourselves. I always thought that was her way of saying not to spend too much on her. But now I understand that it was her way of asking for thoughtful gifts which signified our feelings for her.

I have a very close friend who bakes cupcakes every Christmas. She spends so much time getting the cakes just right, the ingredients all at the correct temperature, the sponge light as a feather and the cakes all symmetrical. Then she ices each one with beautiful buttercream spirals, folds and designs and edible glitter, each one tailored for an individual friend.

She places each one into a pretty box and then walks the roads of north London delivering them by hand. She's walking the dog at the same time, but nevertheless it takes hours.

The thought, care and attention which go into that gift make it so special. Once she's delivered it along with warm hugs, we gather around this cupcake after dinner and split it neatly and ceremoniously into thirds and savour every crumb. I swear it tastes better because it is made with generosity of spirit.

This friend works five days a week for the NHS, has said dog and twins, elderly parents she cares for and a few dozen cakes to deliver. So, I doubly appreciate the effort. Would I prefer a large scented candle from Brunello Cucinelli? Absolutely not.

I'm not proposing we all make collages or crochet a scarf for our nearest and dearest. I *am* suggesting that we put thought and (dare I say it) time into choosing what we give.

Mindful Receiving of Gifts

So now you're on the other side of the present exchange. Someone has placed a gift onto your lap, expectation and hope in their eyes. They're willing you to love this gift. When you open it, you sense that they care. Without wanting to sound too trite, that love and eagerness to bring joy are enough to make the gift special. Many people with fabulous hauls of expensive presents yearn for that abundance of love to be placed on their lap.

How do you reflect that special moment back? How do you show them that they have made you feel loved? Eye contact, awareness of body language and facial expression are all important. Verbally telling them what exactly it is that makes this gift bring you joy shows sincerity.

Whenever you use that shower gel, scented candle or woolly scarf, it's comforting to remember the person who gave it to you with loving kindness, and it means that the gift is not just for that day but for as long as we maintain this practice.

> *Self-absorption in all its forms kills empathy, let alone compassion. When we focus on ourselves, our world contracts as our problems and preoccupations loom large. But when we focus on others, our world expands.*
>
> Daniel Goleman

Pride and Profitability

- Self-focused pride and other-focused pride
- Positive psychology
- Enhancing self-focused pride
- How do I notice the mini-victories?
- Enhancing other-focused pride

> *Happiness is not the absence of problems, it's the ability to deal with them.*
>
> Steven Maraboli

Pride is one of the most meaningful experiences in life.

Self-focused Pride and Other-focused Pride

In the psychology literature, there are numerous studies investigating self-oriented pride, e.g. the pride we get from self-oriented achievements such as passing an exam, placing a central line, repairing a fracture, etc.

In workplace-orientated studies, pride can also be seen as more of a collective attitude derived from team achievements and fostered by the sense of belonging. This is other-focused pride.

This applies to veterinary practices especially. Similar to the feeling the whole team gets after a successful caesarean section where every team member has a puppy, and the surgeon is swelling with geniality while suturing up. Or when we resuscitate a collapsed patient post road traffic accident (RTA) and chest trauma. Or when we, as a team, tend to a client who has many needs and worries.

By looking at this dynamic pride from self and from the team, we can see many opportunities for enhancing pride in ourselves and in the workplace. For discussion, we could further divide pride into self-focused short-term pride, self-focused long-term pride, other-focused short-term pride and other-focused long-term pride.

Most goals will fall into self-focused short-term pride and other-focused long-term pride. For simplicity, let's concentrate on these.

Mental Wellbeing and Positive Psychology for Veterinary Professionals: A Pre-emptive, Proactive and Solution-based Approach, First Edition. Laura Woodward.
© 2024 John Wiley & Sons Ltd. Published 2024 by John Wiley & Sons Ltd.

Positive Psychology

In general, we all feel our work life holds more meaning when we are:

- motivated by cherished goals, e.g. exams, promotions
- aware of self-improvement, e.g. appraisals, more responsibility, etc.
- involved in healthy interpersonal relationships
- loyal to our beliefs and ethics.

It's only recently, with the emergence of what is called positive psychology, that happiness became something we can actually study and even attempt to measure. This new branch of psychology, while it may seem obviously important now, has shifted the research focus from pathology (i.e. analysing personality disorders, psychological pathology and traumas) to optimal human function and flourishing, and it addresses how to enable individuals and work communities to thrive (Seligman 2011).

> Positive psychology has promoted human flourishing as the ultimate goal of scientific research.

That's why counselling is no longer solely something for when you're desperate and in crisis. It's a therapy for *enhancing* wellbeing as well.

There is a massive area of product design dedicated to the development of technology for psychological wellbeing and human potential – so-called 'positive computing'.

The discipline of design has been inspired by the mindset of positive psychology:

- from preventing pain towards promoting happiness (bandages with pictures of teddy bears on them for children)
- from material sufficiency towards experiential value (Pohlmeyer 2012) (alarm clocks that brighten slowly and then burst into birdsong)
- from immediate response towards long-term impact (SAD light visors).

Human flourishing has essentially changed the traditional design process, exemplified by recent scholarly advice, such as 'think experience before product' (Hassenzahl 2010).

So, translating this to the veterinary workplace, humans (the staff) will flourish better and be more productive if they have what is called pride experience in the workplace. Positive psychology promotes enhancing workplace happiness rather than the old-fashioned 'putting out fires' attitude of getting by.

Enhancing Self-focused Pride

Every day at work we do something worthwhile, something worthy of pride. It mightn't be the fracture repair or central line placement mentioned earlier. It may be the swift running of a blood sample, the effective handling of a difficult client interaction, remembering the name of the dog in the waiting room, getting the inappetent patient to eat.

All too often, we don't notice the mini-victories. Why? We're too busy. There's no time for basking in glory. It's only a mini-victory. I do it all the time. I could do that in my sleep.

And yet, all the people who ask you what you do for a living, who gasp in admiration and envy when you tell them, would be over the moon with joy and pride if they were able to take blood and run it, use a feeding tube or take radiographs. It's as though we've become immune to the feeling of achievement once we've achieved a task once. Never to be revisited.

How Do I Notice the Mini-victories?

Mindfulness. Only you can change you.

It takes no time. It's simply focusing on noticing the present moment rather than only noticing the things which need fixing, the next task, the problem list.

If we take a random hour at work, making a conscious decision to notice every small victory in that hour, with your whole attention for as long as is practical, is a great place to start.

At first, it will take a lot of effort and may be quite tiring. With practice, you will notice that a few mini-victories added together make for a good feeling. A few good feelings a day might accumulate to a great day. Noticing several great days a month may be the difference between feeling pride in yourself and leaving the practice.

Enhancing Other-focused Pride

This pride comes from interpersonal interactions and the influence between oneself and others.

Moral accomplishment as an individual and as a team is associated with a feeling of pride and inner wellbeing. We can take intrinsic pride in how we work. This experience of pride can be appreciated and felt by others in our social interactions in the clinic and contribute to our psychological empowerment and promote future successes (Froman 2010). Therefore, it follows that we are uniquely placed to feel other-focused pride during the progression of events from treating the client with care and kindness, to communicating well as a team, to each member of the team enhancing the client experience, diagnosing, treating, discharging and following up. Then placing the thank-you card from the client up on the communal board so we can all feel that same sense of achievement.

Katzenbach (2003) talks about a powerful closed loop of energy derived from pride: 'Better performance contributes to business success, and recognised business success instils a strong feeling of pride, which fuels future better performance'.

It's a no-brainer really. Self-focused pride is something I can achieve today in the next hour. Other-focused pride I can achieve by looking around me at the team and then contributing to the team. Both can grow from there if we make the effort.

References

Froman, L. (2010). Positive psychology in the workplace. *Journal of Adult Development* 17 (2): 59–69.

Hassenzahl, M. (2010). Experience design: technology for all the right reasons. *Synthesis Lectures on Human-Centered Informatics* 3 (1): 1–95.

Katzenbach, J. (2003). *Why Pride Matters More than Money: The Power of the World's Greatest Motivational Force*. New York: Crown Business.

Pohlmeyer, A.E. (2012). Design for happiness. *Interfaces* 92: 8–11.

Seligman, M. (2011). *Flourish: A New Understanding of Happiness, Well-Being-and How to Achieve Them*. Boston: Nicholas Brealey Publishing.

Stubborn Optimism

Stubborn optimism is a conscious decision to have an optimistic mindset in order to make change. Often associated with sustainability and the current climate crisis, stubborn optimism also describes beautifully how we, as tiny individuals in a massive world, can effect change through our behaviour.

I recently chatted with someone whose job it is to show large companies how to be more sustainable, and how to implement changes from tiny adjustments to massive transformations within the company.

Of course, a lot of this is becoming more known due to the climate crisis, and we're hearing more of it in the veterinary world which is hopeful.

Many of this person's co-workers are suffering from despair and poor mental wellbeing where they have to leave their posts. The lack of change they see around them is causing serious mental health concerns in this industry.

We are often in denial about what is happening around us – governments are treading too carefully and making agreements too slowly to keep global warming under 1.5°. That target is long gone. The current trajectory is 3–4° by 2050. Our children will be middle-aged or old when that happens.

And yet wildfires are happening in London, for goodness sake, not just Australia, and the floods, famine, droughts and heatwaves cannot be blamed on one cohort of people, nor the fat cats, nor the aggressors of war.

It's a combination of all things human. It's no wonder these strong, optimistic sustainability experts throw their hands in the air and leave, broken.

The stubborn optimist is the person who sees all this lack of motivation for change, ineffective governments and new oil fields being drilled, and still refuses to give up. It's not something they can teach you in management school. This man's stubborn optimism comes from deep and frequent meditation. It's a personal choice to have this mindset while accepting that climate change is happening and people are being displaced and dying.

Mental Wellbeing and Positive Psychology for Veterinary Professionals: A Pre-emptive, Proactive and Solution-based Approach, First Edition. Laura Woodward.
© 2024 John Wiley & Sons Ltd. Published 2024 by John Wiley & Sons Ltd.

It's his career to limit climate change and yet despite the obstinate and purposeful ignoring of the facts by those who don't want to alter their way of working, he knows that what he does makes a difference and decreases the pace of climate change albeit by a small amount.

I cannot imagine how hard that is to do on a global level or even on a company level. But on an individual level it simply has to be done. Not making change is not an option.

At home, I recycle every tiny bit of cardboard I can, I monitor my fuel and electricity consumption and reduce it, we rarely eat meat. That's not virtue signalling. Because at work, I use 20 plastic syringes per patient, my kit is double bagged in plastic and paper, I'm in full PPE for literally everything. It's the antithesis of what I do at home.

So I feel guilty and a fraud.

I put this to my friend who is the expert on sustainability. We also share a love of meditation and Buddhism. He totally got it. Some plastics aren't as bad as others, he said. I also have to be realistic about what needs to be done at work regarding sterility, of course. Finally, being guilty is one of the first steps towards throwing my hands in the air like others and giving up. Guilt would preclude stubborn optimism from becoming my mindset.

It's easy to feel helpless and it's easy to be in denial. But by tiny actions and changes to our mindset, we can effect change.

Sustainability is not just about the climate. If we can create a more cohesive, kinder community, that is actually part of sustainability, because communities coming together can effect change beyond what we usually expect. Also, the effect of a community is usually more than the sum of the individuals effects.

During the COVID-19 pandemic, many people formed local community groups. We did one for my street. We reminded each other of when the bins were being collected and when it was the local postman's birthday.

But more importantly, we created a local community of support and like-mindedness. The group chat is positive and optimistic. That is an easy thing to do: set the tone when you start the group, and moderate the conversation if it's becoming a bit heated or when it's transforming into a platform for venting anger at the council, etc.

Now we go to the pub together, decorate the street for various festivals and have co-ordinated fireworks on New Year's Eve. Before this group existed, people had been living side by side for 10 years and never actually meeting (such is London).

On a minor sustainability note, when anyone has stuff they no longer use or need, it's donated to the group and we all take what we may use. One neighbour managed to distribute five bags of slate and another pair exchanged a bath for a TV.

By being a stubborn optimist and believing that we can indeed make small changes independently, we can bring about a real collective change in what happens in our society. We have to be brave and stubborn.

While it's true that previous generations should have had the stubborn optimism to effect change, in reality we can forgive them for not being as informed as we are now. We have more capability to effect change than they did and maybe our children will have more ability again. However, we are no longer at a crossroads. We had passed the crossroads by the time the Paris Agreement took place. So we cannot leave it to our children to reverse the changes and we cannot proclaim that it's not our responsibility.

Stubborn optimism doesn't just aim to slow down this speeding train of climate destruction, it aims to grind it to a halt and even reverse some of the changes. It seems impossible to me but 'impossible' does not figure in the mindset of a stubborn optimist.

If everyone had given up 15 years ago, we would be in an even worse climate crisis than we are now. Difficult to imagine that.

It's easy to be overwhelmed when we receive more news every month about how the planet is getting warmer and warmer – the bushfires, the glacial melts, the heatwaves.

It's relentless. And it's frustrating watching our governments behaving like nasty children in the playground instead of effecting change for the environment.

What Can I Do?

We can aim to make small choices in our workplaces every day. It's easy to underestimate the impact of those small choices.

Take an example of one business making the switch to a renewable energy provider. A simple choice like that can be as powerful as 50 households making that decision. So although you may be only one person in that business, you can make a much bigger difference than you could do just in your own personal life.

Perhaps be the person who starts recycling the paper from autoclave bags. Be the person who puts out the idea to use environmentally friendly laundry capsules for the bedding. Be the person to request drugs from the more ethical drugs companies,

Small achievable changes create instant wins that translate into bigger impacts down the line

> Stubborn optimism is about starting anywhere because if you don't start, that's not an option.

We have to start somewhere and feel that momentum. Through that we can actually, over time, compound that impact little by little.

Resilience

- Mindfulness and Resilience
- Positive emotion
- Engagement
- Relationships
- Meaning
- Accomplishments

> *You never know how strong you are until being strong is the only choice you have.*
>
> Bob Marley

Resilience is more than 'bouncing back from adversity'. It's also the ability to avoid becoming overwhelmed by adversity in the first place.

Resilience is a personal trait that helps individuals to cope with trying circumstances and achieve good adjustment and development when life becomes really tough, as it will do.

Life is always changing.

> Everything changes, nothing stays the same, and that can be okay.

Mindfulness and Resilience

Mindfulness, meditation and mindful living help us to avoid ruminating and spiralling into unhelpful ways of thinking, and, instead, to foster solution-based ways of seeing our experiences.

So, resilience in the face of adversity is an obvious benefit of mindfulness because the adversity doesn't give rise to automatic ways of negative thinking and depressogenic rumination. Mindfulness is antecedent to resilience.

Neuroscience shows that mindfulness improves the connections between the emotive prefrontal cortex and the reasoning amygdala. This prevents us from allowing negative experiences to cause a downwards spiralling (Davidson and Begley 2012).

Isn't this what resilience looks like from the outside?

Mental Wellbeing and Positive Psychology for Veterinary Professionals: A Pre-emptive, Proactive and Solution-based Approach, First Edition. Laura Woodward.
© 2024 John Wiley & Sons Ltd. Published 2024 by John Wiley & Sons Ltd.

Indian researchers Bajaj and Pande, writing in the journal *Personality and Individual Differences*, published evidence that mindfulness improves resilience (Bajaj and Pande 2015).

> Mindful people can cope better than others with difficult thoughts and emotions without becoming overwhelmed or shutting down.

Their study includes research correlating better life satisfaction in people who practise mindfulness techniques compared to those who don't. They hypothesise that improved resilience is one of the mediators of this improved overall wellbeing and life satisfaction.

Bajaj and Pande describe a study featuring 327 undergraduates (236 men and 91 women). The students completed a series of surveys measuring their mindfulness, life satisfaction, emotional state and level of resilience. While this study has several limitations, e.g. the results being subjective, the representations of males vs females, etc., we know that measures of mindfulness are associated with higher levels of subjective wellbeing (Wang and Kong 2014, Wenzel et al. 2015).

Some studies with university students proposed mediators such as emotional intelligence, core self-evaluation and self-esteem as being amongst the reasons why our lives improve because of mindfulness. We know that mindfulness improves all of the above.

It was the aim of Bajaj and Pande to prove that resilience is yet another mediator in this correlation.

Another study of 124 firefighters showed that trait mindfulness was negatively related to depressive and PTSD symptoms and alcohol problems, suggesting that trait mindfulness may reduce avoidant coping in response to stress, and contribute to resilience (Smith et al. 2008).

So, mindfulness subconsciously improves resilience and resilience improves mental wellbeing. Fantastic. But how do I use mindfulness to consciously improve my resilience?

As veterinary professionals, not only do we demand the evidence base but we also then need clear instructions on how to do it, ideally as soon as possible (yesterday would be ideal), in as short a time as possible, with the greatest effects. Conveniently, we also love acronyms. So, I introduce you to PERMA.

- Positive emotion
- Engagement

- Relationships
- Meaning
- Accomplishments

Dr Martin Seligmann has devoted his life to the promotion of happiness in people. His PERMA model was designed as a model of contentment, positivity and resilience. Let's take a closer look.

Positive Emotion

This involves nurturing our thought patterns towards a positive outlook. See this section, Chapter 7 on two ways of looking.

If we accept that there are two ways of seeing a situation, often we will choose the more pleasing, positive way. Sometimes we won't, because we don't relate to it or it doesn't sit well with us. Nevertheless, noticing that there is 'another way of looking' gives rise to, at the least, less negative emotions.

Also, choosing where our focus lies through meditation is entirely within our control.

Engagement

This is mindfulness really. Mindful working, mindful living, being present.

Relationships

We aren't always in control of how nurturing and fulfilling our relationships are. But we are in control of how much time and attention we give to our relationships.

Recognising the toxic ones is a key life skill. Getting rid of the life-draining, exhausting, poisonous people in your life will be the decluttering which brings lasting peace and happiness like nothing else.

If you can't avoid some of the toxic people, avoid spending your precious time focusing on them, their social media and their lives.

Use the head space you free up to mindfully observe who brings you real joy. Who is actually good? Who in your life is happy because you're happy?

Who are the people who like peace instead of chaos? People who exude that feeling of positivity, kindness and fun.

Investing your time and energy in those relationships instead of the ones which are detrimental to your wellbeing is a no-brainer.

Meaning

This means having a purpose.

Remember the question 'Can you be so deeply rooted in your purpose that even putting out the bins becomes meaningful?'.

Noticing that everything you do has a purpose and is meaningful enhances your self-worth.

Everything you do, from saving a life, to making a coffee to slobbing in front of the TV, has a purpose.

Accomplishments

Having goals and ambition is great. Being veterinary professionals means that we've already achieved a great deal.

Noticing all the victories, including the mini-victories is essential, and often what has been evading us for so long.

There's no need to berate yourself for underachieving; there are plenty of people in life who'll do that job for you.

Returning to Bajaj and Pande's questionnaire, mindfulness – or a lack thereof – was measured by their responses to 15 assertions, such as 'I tend to walk quickly to get where I'm going without paying attention to what I experience along the way'.

To gauge their resilience, participants were presented with 10 self-descriptive statements, including 'able to adapt to change', 'can stay focused under pressure' and 'not easily discouraged by failure'. They responded to each on a five-point scale ('not at all' to 'true nearly all of the time').

As predicted, the researchers found that 'individuals with higher mindfulness have greater resilience, thereby increasing their life satisfaction'. They note that resilience 'can be seen as an important source of subjective well-being', and point out many ways in which mindfulness can promote this state of mind.

'Mindful people can better cope with difficult thoughts and emotions without becoming overwhelmed or shutting down (emotionally)', they write. 'Pausing and observing the mind may help us to resist getting drawn into wallowing in a setback.'

Put another way, mindfulness 'weakens the chain of associations that keep people obsessing about' their problems or failures, which increases the likelihood they will try again.

'The findings provide support for universities to develop strategies that promote mindfulness', Bajaj and Pande conclude. 'Mindfulness training could provide a practical means of enhancing resilience, and personality characteristics like optimism, zest, and patience.'

References

Bajaj, B. and Pande, N. (2015). Mediating role of resilience in the impact of mindfulness on life satisfaction and affect as indices of subjective well-being. *Personality and Individual Differences* 93: 63–67.

Davidson, R.J. and Begley, S. (2012). *The Emotional Life of Your Brain: How Its Unique Patterns Affect the Way You Think, Feel, and Live – and How You Can Change Them*. New York: Hudson Street Press.

Smith, B.W., Dalen, J., Wiggins, K. et al. (2008). The Brief Resilience Scale: assessing the ability to bounce back. *International Journal of Behavioral Medicine* 15 (3): 194–200.

Wang, K. and Kong, F. (2014). Linking trait mindfulness to life satisfaction in adolescents: the mediating role of resilience and self-esteem. *Child Indicators Research* 13: 321–335.

Wenzel, M., von Versen, C., Hirschmüller, S., and Kubiak, T. (2015). Curb your neuroticism – mindfulness mediates the link between neuroticism and subjective wellbeing. *Personality and Individual Differences* 80: 68–75.

Two Ways of Looking

Try this exercise. Look at the main headline on your news app. Although being non-judgemental is what we're ultimately aiming for, we are human and we will have various thoughts when it comes to world events and local news.

Without much contemplation, say the first reaction you have out loud. It might be 'That's terrible' or 'She's a monster' or 'Thank goodness'. (Although these days, news corporations seem to only headline atrocities to engage our natural negativity bias. And it works.)

Back to the exercise. Now try to imagine another person reading the same headlines and having a different reaction from you; for example, 'People will have to be resilient' or 'I wonder what goes through her mind' or 'Some people won't like that as much as I do', etc.

Basically, this exercise shows us that there is always another way to look at something, contrary to our views and feelings.

The point of the exercise is not to persuade you, or me, to feel differently about a person, event or situation. Our initial reaction is our initial reaction. Rather, the point is that looking at situations from two differing ways softens the effect that situation has on us. It opens us up to other people's points of view which are in contrast to our own and makes us better conversationalists and better listeners.

It challenges our automatic, reflexive, deeply held views which can stimulate us into thought and self-questioning in a gentle curious way.

It can be fascinating to look inside your own mind and enquire why you feel the way you do. Like a healthy debate between two kind people.

When things are tough, this is definitely not about 'turning that frown upside down'. Sometimes this exercise can be nearly impossible. However, the more difficult it is, the more effective it is. It's interesting to practise this exercise several times a day, with anything. Even if someone else is loving the glorious sunshine, you might be too hot. Elton John's last show at Glastonbury may be a time of sadness for some and of celebration for others. Soup being hot might be warming for one person and too hot to eat quickly for another. Notice what effect it has on you.

Mental Wellbeing and Positive Psychology for Veterinary Professionals: A Pre-emptive, Proactive and Solution-based Approach, First Edition. Laura Woodward.
© 2024 John Wiley & Sons Ltd. Published 2024 by John Wiley & Sons Ltd.

'Love thine enemy' is a phrase that appears in many religious belief systems. For most of us, that is beyond what we even want to do. It feels inappropriate and false to force myself to even like a person who lies, cheats, abuses, gaslights, steals, etc.

I took this question to my mentor, a Sri Lankan Buddhist monk, with an air of 'Don't be ridiculous. I'm not doing that'.

He persuaded me to try, in the safety of my own meditation, to at least be sure not to hate. That can take effort in many cases.

If we can move from hating to not hating, then trying to extend that to at least accepting that the person we are visualising is a weak, fellow human being with many faults and flaws, this takes the fire out of our bitterness and that is a more peaceful way to feel than being full of bad will.

Trying to focus on this 'bad' person not so much with pity but rather with a type of compassion where we wish them more peace than they have at the moment would be good (people who cause harm to us are not content, ever).

Instead of relishing the fact that they act out of a deep misery within them, it is good to move to just observing that they are deeply unsatisfied and in turmoil. Forcing yourself to wish them less turmoil will not negate your feelings and it will not put you in more danger of being hurt by them again.

It will, however, bring you some relief. At least try it.

How Mindfulness Can Improve Cardiac Health

> Depression predicts the excess risk of developing coronary heart disease or myocardial infarction by a whopping 30%.

The husband of one of the teachers shot dead in the 2022 Texas school massacre in Uvalde died of a heart attack two days later, overcome with grief.

Stress cardiomyopathy, commonly referred to as 'broken heart syndrome', can cause the heart to fail as a result of extreme grief, emotional distress or surprise. The risk of heart attack increases 21-fold within 24 hours after the loss of a loved one (Mostofsky et al. 2012).

While this is an extreme example of horrifically negative emotions leading to cardiac failure, we did already know that difficult emotions risk harming the heart.

For example, a 2014 meta-analysis of 30 prospective studies (40 independent reports), with 893 850 participants and follow-ups ranging from two to 37 years, found that depression predicted the excess risk of developing coronary heart disease or myocardial infarction by a whopping 30% (Gan et al. 2014).

Post-traumatic stress disorder, anxiety, anger, frustration and unrelenting job stress all pose similar cardiovascular risks, and probably share a common physiological pathway.

So, why am I telling you this when you may have been feeling good about life? Because the converse is also true and that is very good news indeed.

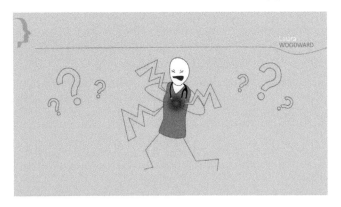

Cultivating positive emotions like gratitude, empathy and compassion can give rise to a better cardiac state and create a circle of decreased stress and more calm. This is especially helpful for those of us who worry and stress about our health.

In one large trial, 97 253 healthy women were followed for over eight years. Optimists were found to have a lower risk of CHD (chronic heart disease), including 30% lower CHD mortality, and 14% lower total mortality. Those with higher levels of cynicism and hostility were found to have a higher risk of early death, either from cancer or other causes (Tindle et al. 2009). The mechanisms can be indirect, which many would feel is obvious. But there are direct effects also.

Pessimism and cynical hostility may affect the risks of physical disease via two main pathways: directly, by altering activation of the autonomic nervous system, hypothalamic-pituitary axis or other stress response systems, which may in turn speed up the process of diseases such as atherosclerosis; and indirectly, by influencing health behaviours such as drinking excessively, vaping, smoking and poor eating habits.

In the study by Tindle et al., the magnitude of the effects of optimism and cynical hostility was similar to the effect of hypertension for total mortality.

The fact that these psychological factors are modifiable increases their clinical relevance. If we change the way we behave and react, if we choose to live life more meaningfully and more calmly, we can literally save it. What better incentive could there be than to live a longer and healthier life?

Many of us already knew that people with a personality commonly referred to as 'Type A' have a higher risk of developing heart disease than others. Most vets and many nurses fall into that Type A category. However, thankfully, more recent studies have shown that it's only certain traits in this cohort that increase cardiovascular disease risk. For example, angry and hostile Type A people, anxious Type A people and narcissistic Type A people are all at increased risk of developing heart disease, as are Type A people with depression.

It follows that, by learning new ways of behaving and therefore new ways of being, we can use neuroplasticity to our advantage when it comes to cardiac health and longevity.

Emotions are the precursor of feelings. They originate in the limbic centres of the brain (the amygdala). This information is transferred to the reasoning and planning centres in the prefrontal cortex, giving rise to feelings.

Antonio Damasio, chair in neuroscience, as well as professor of psychology, philosophy and neurology at the University of Southern California, says that feelings are the meanings which we give to our emotions. These meanings are usually based on previous experiences and memories.

For example, the emotion of alertness on hearing a door slam shut might elicit a feeling of fear in one person if they grew up in a household where someone repeatedly slammed doors in anger. This feeling then may be accompanied by rapid heart rate, hypertension and hypercoagulability along with other physical symptoms of fear.

However, someone else who grew up in a stable household, with parents in control of their reactions to emotions (emotional intelligence), might have that same emotion of alertness on hearing the door slam shut but in contrast, they would be more likely to progress to the feeling of curiosity and wonder about where the wind was coming from which caused the door to slam, or who had just come home.

The effects of our anger and rage on our children's mental health have been briefly touched upon in Part Three, Chapter 16 on anger. Now, we can see that we also have a moral responsibility to be mindful of the effects of our out-of-control emotions on our children's future cardiac health as well as their mental health.

References

Gan, Y., Gong, Y., Tong, X. et al. (2014). Depression and the risk of coronary heart disease: a meta-analysis of prospective cohort studies. *BMC Psychiatry* 14: Article number 371.

Mostofsky, E., Maclure, M., Sherwood, J. et al. (2012). Risk of acute myocardial infarction after the death of a significant person in one's life. The Determinants of Myocardial Infarction Onset Study. *Circulation* 125: 491–496.

Tindle, H., Chang, Y., Kuller, L. et al. (2009). Optimism, cynical hostility, and incident coronary heart disease and mortality in the Women's Health Initiative. *Circulation* 120: 656–662.

Self-compassion Versus Self-care

- Mindfulness
- Loving kindness towards yourself
- Hand-on-heart meditation
- A sense of common humanity

> Taking care of myself doesn't mean 'me first', it means 'me too'.

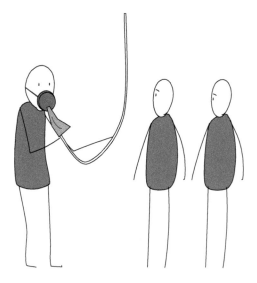

We've made the analogy of putting your own oxygen mask on first so that you can help others with theirs. Self-care is so important if we are to maintain a stable mindset during challenging times and to be a source of strength and happiness for others.

The three components of self-compassion are *Mindfulness*, which helps with self-awareness in a balanced way, *Loving kindness towards ourselves*, which means that we need to cultivate a strong motivation to relieve our suffering, and *A sense of common humanity*, which means taking some solace from the fact that we are not alone in our experiences and feelings.

Mental Wellbeing and Positive Psychology for Veterinary Professionals: A Pre-emptive, Proactive and Solution-based Approach, First Edition. Laura Woodward.
© 2024 John Wiley & Sons Ltd. Published 2024 by John Wiley & Sons Ltd.

Self-compassion is more than just self-care. When we are truly self-compassionate, we relate to our feelings in an accepting manner to defuse their hold on us.

It is often said that we should treat others the way we would wish them to treat us. I propose treating *ourselves* the way we would want others to treat us – so how would you treat a friend who is struggling, and how can you extend that effort towards yourself? Do you find yourself desperate for a coffee and then, when you get it, slugging it down while typing your notes frantically? Do you run yourself a bath and then spend your time in it scrolling through your long list of emails? Do you wonder why, if you are exercising self-care by making yourself a coffee and running a bath, you're not feeling the benefits of it?

Ask yourself this. If a friend were struggling, anxious and exhausted, would you place a cup of coffee in their hand and then walk away, job done? Would you sit them in a comfortable seat and then scroll through your emails, ignoring them? No, of course, you wouldn't. So why do we do this to ourselves?

Why do we pay so little attention to ourselves and think that the material external aspects of self-care are enough to 'fix' us? Why does looking after ourselves and offering loving kindness to ourselves end up on the long list of chores we really don't have time for? So, we half-heartedly do it to 'get it done'.

You may have children, colleagues and clients all depending on you to help them, and it's difficult not to experience emotional fatigue. This state of sympathetic overdrive can send us on a downward spiral into a state where we are no good to anyone.

Taking time out to stabilise and recharge is essential if we are to survive. Ironically, keeping our heads just above water by running a bath and hoping that'll be enough, for now, is simply not enough.

Let's look at the three elements of self-compassion.

Mindfulness

Mindfulness helps with self-awareness in a balanced way. As we know, mindfulness is focusing on the present moment on purpose, as if your life depended on it. And yet, focusing on the present moment, when it's full of difficulties, seems counterproductive. However, avoiding feeling what you're feeling, in order to feel it a bit less, will allow those emotions to grow into something truly unmanageable before they come back to haunt you at a later time. So, we need to deal with them as they happen.

It's easy to ruminate and to get lost in the drama especially when the current situation is so overwhelming. Mindfulness helps us to relate to what we are feeling in an accepting manner. For example, 'I feel anxious that the pressures of work will be too enormous for me to bear'.

Rather than analysing the anxiety and its origins, instead of justifying it, instead of judging it, simply accepting that anxiety is the thing I'm feeling, and allowing myself to feel it, can defuse the hold that it has on me.

Have you ever noticed that sometimes, when you talk about what's upsetting you to a friend, they immediately begin a sentence with 'well, at least' or 'never mind' or even 'it could be worse'?

This is a genuine effort by a kind friend to help you, but active listening doesn't respond with unhelpful comments. Active listening means being there in the moment with your friend, silently understanding, pausing to digest what they've said, relating on a deep level to what they're expressing. True empathy doesn't sweep your friend's uncomfortable feelings under the carpet in an effort to jolly them up. No, we pause, reflect and share the load by staying quiet.

So, can you do that for yourself? When you make yourself that coffee or run that bath, can you then spare yourself the time to just be there with yourself at that moment? Like you would with a friend in need. Truly listening instead of scrolling through your messages. Accepting and understanding that it hurts. Taking the time to just be and to breathe.

Loving Kindness Towards Yourself

What does this mean? We need to cultivate a strong motivation to relieve our own suffering. It's vitally important. You can make it okay for you. You can make it better than okay for you.

But it needs to be deeper than just physical wellbeing if it's going to weather the ongoing difficulties of a normal human life. It needs to be hand-on-heart meditations and more.

Hand-on-heart Meditation

Hold your right hand on your heart as if to say to yourself 'I'm here for you'. Like a close friend offering comfort. Close your eyes. Taking normal breaths, concentrate only on the in-breath for a while. Imagine you are breathing in strength, loving kindness and calm. Imagine it as a valve mechanism and the in-breaths are 'inflating' the inner wellbeing. Every in-breath adds to the strength, love and calm inside you. Feel the solace growing inside of you.

When you feel a calm, warm sensation within, when you are fully 'inflated', stay focused on it for as long as is comfortable.

A Sense of Common Humanity

By this, I mean taking some solace from the fact that we are not alone in our experiences and feelings. Suffering is part of the human experience but knowing that we are not alone can help to ease the added anxiety. Noticing this is another act of self-compassion.

Treat yourself as you would wish others to treat you.

Being Ready for Some Good News

- Why we tend to ignore the good moments
- Three practices to help us notice the good news

I got my teen and preteen out of bed this morning at dawn. That was after clearing up kitten diarrhoea, medicating the other cat, putting back into the bins that which the foxes had strewn all over the road, packing lunches, shoving some sort of food into myself, triaging the day's necessities, organising the ops list at work. Mindlessly.

My daughter called out for me. Had I forgotten the PE kit? Was she worried about school? Whatever the problem, I'd just have to sort it and get to work.

No. She had looked out the window, seen a pink sunrise and paused to appreciate it. Then she had shared that moment, describing the trees being silhouetted like palm trees on an exotic island. And it felt good.

Her delight was refreshing. And a reminder to me to practise what I preach.

Yes, we have worldwide viruses causing death and misery. We are under the constant threat of major powers being at war, earthquakes and floods are taking countless lives and displacing millions of people. What's happening is overwhelming if we allow it to be overwhelming. But it's also in her life. Being a child doesn't shield you from the news. But being child-like in allowing ourselves to take a good moment and make it huge and very present is a talent we can learn from those to whom we often preach.

It takes effort. We do have to coax these small moments of joy into our awareness. And then hold them there for longer than our autopilot-minds would comfortably do. Because being realistic, the bigger picture is fairly grim these days. If we can shrink our attention right down to the mundane but pleasant experiences just a few times a day, and revel in the joy they bring, then that joy becomes bigger.

I'm not suggesting we pretend that we're anywhere other than on this planet. That would be a denial of the truth. It's just hopping off the hamster wheel of life for a moment several times a day and saying 'Stop' to

Mental Wellbeing and Positive Psychology for Veterinary Professionals: A Pre-emptive, Proactive and Solution-based Approach, First Edition. Laura Woodward.
© 2024 John Wiley & Sons Ltd. Published 2024 by John Wiley & Sons Ltd.

ourselves. Stop and look/smell/taste the mundane good things and try to make them mundane *great* things which take up five minutes of our day instead of a fleeting five seconds.

Why We Tend to Ignore the Good Moments

Even without a pandemic or global disaster weighing on us, human beings tend to be downcast. The brain registers negative experiences more strongly than positive ones because it helped our ancestors to survive. It's useful to have a brain highly attuned to threats when sabre-toothed tigers lurk in the darkness.

It's far less helpful when threats to our physical survival are fewer, and when our enduring desire is to be at ease.

We have evolved and we have developed so many methods of making our lives safer and our lifestyles convenient and luxurious. What's the point of inventing the wheel and building roads to make life more convenient if we allow the traffic jams to irritate us as much as travelling on foot irritated our ancestors?

Paying attention to joyful moments takes practice. When we learnt mindful meditation and how to pay attention, on purpose, to the present moment, it was learning to pay attention *no matter what the moment*, even if it is a dreadful moment. So surely, paying attention to a pleasant moment should be easier?

Not necessarily. It's pulling against our minds which are naturally hard-wired to move on from the pleasant and safe good moments to more 'important' things.

Soaking in moments of delight requires mindfulness. It's challenging, for example, to enjoy the fact that the cat's bloods are normal when you're doom-scrolling on Twitter.

Three Practices to Help Us Notice the Good News

Shift Your Frame of Reference

So often, we reserve celebration for milestones – a wedding day, the birth of a child or a hard-won promotion. When we think of joy as belonging only to big events, we side-line the many small pleasures strewn along the way. Finding joy in the small things makes it far more accessible and creates a positive feedback loop. The more we attend to joy in the ordinary moments of our lives, the more we experience it and the more joyous we become.

Living More Mindfully

We talked about slowing down just a tad in order to notice. Noticing the small pleasures will be easier if we make an effort to be living and doing in the present moment. Right now, you're reading this. Try to put other thoughts, actions and phone pinging out of your mind. Take a moment to just be.

Noticing What's Not Wrong

Sometimes it can be as simple as savouring the moment when you do have time for three deep breaths because no one's bleeding and no one's crying.

Maybe make a list of what's not wrong. For example, the house isn't flooded, I don't have a headache, the car starts, the dog didn't throw up and I have a coffee in my hand.

> *Knowing you are not entirely at the mercy of agitation can bring some joy.*
>
> Chade-Meng Tan

The Use of Language

- Internal monologue
- External words to self
- External words to others

Internal monologue and external words can have a profound effect on our own mental wellbeing and on the wellbeing of others. By pausing to choose our language carefully, and with the help of emotional intelligence skills, we can enhance the communal mood.

> *Don't mix bad words with your bad mood. You'll have many opportunities to change a mood, but you'll never get the opportunity to replace the words you spoke.*
>
> Unknown

A truly eloquent friend of mine recently asked me 'Have you noticed how many people describe being stuck in traffic as a "disaster", or spilling a cup of coffee as a "mess" or (the big one) a case going wrong as "devastating"? Well, how's about being stuck in traffic is a "nuisance", spilling your coffee is a "pain" and an unsuccessful case is a "disappointment"!'

His words made me think. If we make the effort to ensure that our internal monologue is helpful and constructive (or at least non-damaging), then that's one less person bringing us down, and also our external words will be helpful and constructive for others.

Internal Monologue

Psychologists reckon that only about one in 10 of us *don't* have chatter going on in our head for most of the day. It might be a list of things to do, an email we're composing, a conversation we want to have or wished we'd had, anything.

So what a fantastic opportunity this is to speak kindly to ourselves and to choose our language carefully.

Mental Wellbeing and Positive Psychology for Veterinary Professionals: A Pre-emptive, Proactive and Solution-based Approach, First Edition. Laura Woodward.
© 2024 John Wiley & Sons Ltd. Published 2024 by John Wiley & Sons Ltd.

I rarely swear out loud. But internally, when I drop and smash something, inadvertently lock myself out of the house or spill tea on my laptop, my internal monologue is the stuff of nightmares.

However, if my friend does the same or if my kids break plates or the cat spills a pint of water on my electronics, I use calm, reassuring words and tone of voice, because it's a simple mistake and they may be distressed already.

So why the disparity?

We've talked before about treating yourself as you would treat a friend. A helpful practice is to choose the words for our internal monologue as carefully as we would choose words for a friend or our child. Before long, it becomes a habit, so choosing helpful words and phrases for our external voice becomes something we do automatically. As a massive added benefit, the less internal self-flagellation we practise, the better our self-esteem and confidence.

External Words to Self

There's little benefit in being attentive to our use of language towards others and congratulating ourselves on our kindness if we call ourselves an 'idiot' out loud for forgetting something or if we swear at ourselves when we drop coffee on the carpet.

More damaging than the coffee stain on the carpet is the effect it has on our children and loved ones to hear us berate ourselves if we do it out loud. How can they have healthy self-esteem and feel unjudged if their role model is cursing their own simple mistakes?

External Words to Others

If you have high levels of emotional intelligence, what you say can be profoundly powerful to those around you and to yourself.

Emotional intelligence has the five key elements: self-awareness, self-regulation, motivation, empathy and social skills. We should ideally be putting all of these into practice each and every time we open our mouths.

With practice, you can run through all these in a few milliseconds.

- *Self-awareness*: how do I feel?
- *Self-regulation*: am I going to speak to myself or to someone else reactively or after some thought?

- *Motivation*: what do I want to achieve out of this situation?
- *Empathy*: am I aware of how the other person feels? What type of language will resonate with them? Cognitive empathy is, after all, about using the language of the other person rather than our own.
- *Social skills*: what tone and volume do I need to use in order to achieve my goal? Is my body language going to reflect what I want to say and how I want to say it?

Let's take a (potentially unhelpful) everyday situation and apply emotionally intelligent use of language to it.

Driving to work in London traffic can be many different things to different people. For some, it's a daily, boring, time-wasting source of stress which always takes longer than expected. For others, it's a chilled alternative to the tube, with music or guided meditation playing, a good coffee in the holder and a chance to take deep breaths.

Someone cuts in front of me from the lane that was for turning right only, then stops while they catch up on their phone.

Self-awareness: how do I feel? Angry? Enraged? Vengeful? Nonplussed? Amused? Or can I take it to the next level and say 'Thank you' to this driver for helping me to exercise my patience? Seriously, every time I try this, I smile.

No emotion is right or wrong. You don't need to justify why you are feeling it. The exercise is to notice the emotion and put a name on it rather than be carried away by it.

Self-regulation: I could swear internally or externally. I can sit on the horn. I can tailgate that driver for the next mile. I can shrug. I can smile. I can use any words reactively ranging from 'bloody idiot' to 'meh, whatever'.

> *Between stimulus and response there is a space. In that space lies our power to choose our response. In our response lies our growth and our freedom.*
>
> Viktor E. Frankl

Motivation: here's the thing. I do want to get to work as smoothly and as quickly as possible (and probably in as stress-free a way as possible). So, in my experience, shouting and tailgating rarely result in a driver like that moving faster for me or letting me go in front of them because they can sense that I'm in a hurry.

Also, while it may feel that expressing anger and rage will make the stress go away, basic physiology tells us that that's a fallacy.

So, our internal monologue can be littered with expletives. Try it and monitor your heart rate. Or you can really thank the other driver for helping you to exercise your patience, (comical though it may be), notice the breath, lower your shoulders and see if you can lower your heart rate through deep breaths alone.

In reality, if you get to your destination one car-length slower than intended, that's probably 'just fine'. Your stress levels are going to be way more significant than the time at the end of the journey.

Empathy: cognitive empathy, we know, is about communication whereas emotional empathy is about relating to how the other person is feeling. So, tailgating this individual will resonate with them because that's the language they speak, and will effectively communicate that you're up for this game of caffeine-fuelled aggression.

The converse is also true: by not engaging, and not communicating via words or otherwise, your goal of getting to work in a chilled state is more likely to happen. Using your internal monologue of 'no problem', 'meh', 'thank you', etc. can help you to achieve this state.

Social skills: body language is not just for the benefit of the onlooker. It goes without saying that aggressive gestures out the window are unhelpful. Also unhelpful is colourful internal monologue describing the characteristics of this driver

A quick body scan where you sit up straight, lower your shoulders, relax your face and jaw and breathe, calms you while communicating to roadhogs that your intentions are different from theirs.

An inner monologue of 'yeah, okay, whatever' might fit the bill.

But if thought corrupts language, language can also corrupt thought.
George Orwell

Exercise and Work–Life Balance

- Mindful versus mindless exercise – your call
- Lacking in motivation? Find an exercise you actually like

The term 'work–life balance' implies that work is 'bad' and life outside work is 'good', and that we should try to balance the bad with the good. In fact, the lines are quite blurred between being in the practice and our life outside the workplace. Veterinary medicine is a vocation, a way of life. Not many of us truly forget about work the moment we leave the premises to go home.

And many of us continue to perceive exercise or gym membership as a luxury – an activity we'd *like* to do if only we had more time. While exercise is a form of self-compassion, it should never be a guilty pleasure.

Instead of viewing exercise as something selfish we do for ourselves – a personal indulgence that takes us away from our work – it's time we started considering physical activity as part of the work itself.

Mindful versus Mindless Exercise – Your Call

Vybar Cregan-Reid, a nephew of champion Irish marathon runner Jim Hogan, travelled the world in search of the reasons why people run. He loathes treadmills in the gym, calling them the equivalent of exercise junk food. 'If you want to rescue some of your life from oblivion, stay off the treadmill', he warns.

Some people love the monotony of the treadmill. It can be a place to 'switch off', to exercise without really noticing, a form of mindlessness. If that works for you, brilliant.

Another form of exercise where we 'switch off' and focus only on the activity itself may be tennis, football or rugby. Mindless exercise and escapism are like stepping off the chaotic groundhog day of life for an hour for a breather while getting fit at the same time. Even as a mindfulness practitioner, I totally get that. And I do it regularly.

Others will benefit cognitively so much better by exercising in a *mindful* way, i.e. by exercising and acutely noticing their bodies, their breath, their surroundings.

Mental Wellbeing and Positive Psychology for Veterinary Professionals: A Pre-emptive, Proactive and Solution-based Approach, First Edition. Laura Woodward.
© 2024 John Wiley & Sons Ltd. Published 2024 by John Wiley & Sons Ltd.

For those of you who run outdoors, maybe try this simple task: turn off the music and listen to yourself breathe (or gasp), feel the surface beneath your feet and notice it more than ever before, really look at your surroundings and pay attention, observe every different shade of green you run past, appreciate your ability to run, breathe and be more alive than when on the sofa. This is mindful running as opposed to mindless running.

Lacking in Motivation? Find an Exercise You Actually Like

The essential message here is to find exercise which you enjoy (be it mindlessly or mindfully) and enjoy it as much as possible each and every time you do it. If you perceive it as a chore, not only will the mental benefits be so much less, but you are more likely to give it up at the first sign of a strained quad. It's a no-brainer that you are more likely to stick with something if it's enjoyable.

A 2015 article by Carolina Werle suggests that the framing of physical activity biases subsequent snacking.

> The findings showed that when physical activity was perceived as fun (e.g., when it is labelled as a scenic walk rather than an exercise walk), people subsequently consume less dessert at mealtime and consume fewer hedonic snacks. Engaging in a physical activity seems to trigger the search for reward when individuals perceive it as exercise but not when they perceive it as fun.

Apart from introducing me to the term 'hedonic snack' which, as a chocolate lover, I found a bit disturbing, it demonstrated the link between enjoyable exercise and enjoyable guilt-free eating. Because no dessert or chocolate should be a 'sin' or a 'reward'. How can we really enjoy it if we label sugar like this? Chocolate is chocolate. Exercise is fun so we need no reward for doing it.

Regardless of how you go about incorporating exercise into your routine, reframing it as part of your job makes it a lot easier to make time for it. Remember, you're not abandoning work. On the contrary, you're ensuring that the hours you put in have more value because you have the physical fitness and mental wellbeing to work to a higher standard.

Reference

Werle, C., Wansink, B., and Payne, C. (2015). Is it fun or exercise? The framing of physical activity biases subsequent snacking. *Marketing Letters* 26: 691–702.

Learning from Our Pets

- Lesson one – the importance of a good routine
- Lesson two – feel what I need to feel when I need to feel it
- Lesson three – how to be truly present

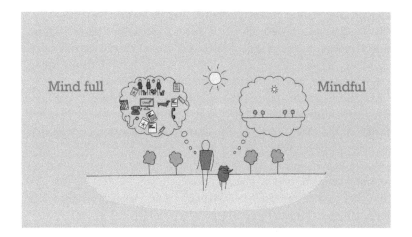

Have you noticed how it seems that everyone, literally everyone, has got a new puppy/kitten/pair of guinea pigs since the COVID-19 pandemic started? While this raises many questions about morals and ethics, it also shows how the human–animal bond can be a lifeline during difficult times.

Looking at the ever increasing number of puppy-poodle crosses amongst my friends and coming through the door at work, I can be either judgemental about pet breeding, grumpy about the fact that work is busier than ever *or* I can choose to celebrate the human–animal bond which has helped me as a pet owner and many, many others to cope with potentially overwhelming emotions related to the pandemic and other massive life challenges It's a choice.

The pandemic normalised the concept of working from home for many. Employers were forced to trust employees to be productive when working away from the office, and to let go of the presumption that it meant a duvet day for them. Most were pleasantly surprised/shocked that working from home, which is evolving into hybrid working for many, not only kept productivity going but for many employees meant an improved work ethic, better mood and, ironically, an increased bond to the firm.

With hybrid working, people describe an excitement they feel on the days when they go in to work and see their co-workers. This has improved team bonding with minimal effort from management.

Office premises have become smaller and therefore less expensive. Most importantly, the quality of life of millions of people has improved. These people can now own a dog, alternate work days with their partners if they have one, spend more time with their kids after school.

And the dogs? They are so 'un-neglected' with hybrid working owners that they are supremely happy (apart from when separated from the owners at the clinic). Yes, behavioural issues have arisen because they are never alone but which bit do you choose to focus on?

Have you ever noticed how, when you're thinking of buying a particular brand or model of car, wherever you look, you keep seeing that car? That's because of unconscious bias: you've subconsciously trained your brain to notice that car.

In a similar way, during mindful meditation, we can consciously train our brain to notice things. For example, how a puppy brought joy into a locked-down family despite the horrors of the pandemic. How my friend's horrible diagnosis has helped those of us around her to come together as a team of support. How concentrating on a good coffee makes its aroma, taste and temperature so much more prominent than normal.

Psychologist Abraham Maslow said, 'If the only tool you have is a hammer, everything looks like a nail'. The more you hold onto a particular belief, the greater the power it has over you.

Simply said, you can literally choose to rejoice in the good things about, for example, increased pet ownership in the UK while being equally aware of the benefits and drawbacks. It's about noticing both, and then choosing which one has the most influence on you.

In an online survey of long-term dog owners in the UK in June 2022, 61% said they found more comfort in their pet than in their fellow human beings (ouch!). Delving further, I can see how their pets, and mine, can have such a profoundly positive effect on us during difficult times.

With that in mind, I'm thinking about what we can learn from our patients and pets.

Lesson One – The Importance of a Good Routine

When we were children, most of us had routines provided for us. We had a wake-up time, school schedules, dinner times and most nights a set bedtime. As much as we complained about those routines, they kept us on a productive path.

Now, as working adults, our routine can be quite dull and monotonous – get up, work, eat, sleep, repeat.

Somewhere in the middle are the dogs and cats: super-chilled bundles of joy on legs who love a routine of walkies, food, nap, repeat (or food, nap, food, nap, food, repeat for the cats).

We can learn from our pets in many ways, and one way is by having an easy routine to add a bit of structure to the days when our default mode is to doom scroll endlessly through the news and social media in search of some relief from world disasters and never finding that relief.

A simple self-care routine can bring some structure to a monotonous, life-draining working week. But 'simple' is the key word. Mindful mini-meditation, mindful shower, slow coffee is an example. Run, bake, achieve, multitask, post on FB, Insta, And BeReal all before 10 a.m. isn't.

Lesson Two – Feel What I Need to Feel When I Need to Feel It

Animals are lucky. Their brain doesn't take them off on a tangent. They don't ruminate in a psychological way like we do. They ruminate physically in such a gorgeous mindful way. For dogs, it's hunger, eat, done. Excitement, walkies, done. Separation anxiety, owner returns, anxiety forgotten. We, however, need to put a whole lot more effort into 'notice, feel, let go' of difficult emotions. It comes with practice.

Environmental disasters, wars and viral pandemics affect more than just our physical health; they tax our mental health as well.

Fear can be at an extremely high level even if it's subliminal. Fear of illness, of loss, of nuclear weaponry, of financial decline – all these are understandable. The non-stop media coverage of news-grabbing morbid headlines and prolonged uncertainty can potentially lead to intense feelings of stress, anxiety and depression. Now more than ever, it's essential for us to create awareness of our feelings and to learn to manage them.

We need to take time out to sit, breathe and allow ourselves to feel what we feel. It's hard to know what we're feeling when it's jumbled up in our minds like a bundle of intertwined wires behind the TV. The very simple act of untangling those wires and sorting them out is so satisfying. As is the act of identifying our feelings, one at a time, and giving each one a name. By naming it, we are identifying each feeling and thus 'allowing' ourselves to feel it.

> It's not weak to feel overwhelmed. It's not selfish to feel sad when others may be worse off. It's not shameful to feel joy when there is a war going on.

Just because I feel overwhelmed + sad + scared, this doesn't preclude the fact that I am also feeling happy to stroke the guinea pigs, play with the kittens, walk the dog.

You are allowed to feel all those emotions. You need to give yourself permission to feel each of those feelings, all the while recognising each individual feeling and emotion as a separate emotion rather than all of them being mashed together as a plethora of intertwined emotions causing anxiety.

As discussed in previous chapters, identifying an emotion doesn't mean you 'become' that emotion. In other words, noticing the feeling is necessary, but getting carried away into a pattern of unhelpful thoughts as a result of the emotion isn't.

It's a subtle difference until you become use to doing it. Notice the emotion, don't become it. Notice the feeling of helplessness while helping yourself to be strong by facing that emotion and thus defusing its hold over you.

Lesson Three – How to Truly Be Present

Just as animals can teach us to let go of difficult emotions (notice they're not 'blocking out' the emotions), they can also show us how to be truly present.

Remember Jon Kabat-Zinn's explanation of mindfulness as being focused on the present moment, non-judgementally, as if our lives depended on it. What dog is yearning for life to return to the way it was when they were young while they're out for a walk? What kitten is yearning for the financial markets to stabilise so they can plan for the future while they're playing with a ping pong ball? The simplicity of their minds allows them to notice the present moment wholeheartedly. And it brings them fun and joy.

When times are hard, really hard like when my mother had just died in front of me, it's impossible to be anywhere else other than totally consumed in the moment of awful grief and desolation.

So, when times are pleasant enough, or even really good, why does it take such effort to remain in that moment and glean all the happiness possible out of it to provide future resilience? It just does. Because we have hard-wired ourselves to ignore things which don't need 'fixing'. It takes training to change. It takes practice. And it's so incredibly rewarding.

So, if we are going to achieve anything during the difficult times, maybe it could be to *develop a simple routine* whereby we allow ourselves the *time to feel what we feel* and *be totally present* in the moment we're in. Because the past has passed and cannot be changed or undone and the future is overwhelmingly uncertain.

If our pets and patients can do it, so can we.

Resolutions and Intentions and Mindfulness-based Eating Awareness Therapy

In making our New Year resolutions, we are setting ourselves goals which we want to achieve. Nothing harmful in that. The danger lies in how we are lining ourselves up for failure and the self-flagellation which ensues.

New Year *intentions* differ from New Year *resolutions*. It's not just semantics.

An intention to do something makes it more achievable despite the gentler phrase. Unlike resolutions, which are tied to a specific outcome and can be more prone to failure, intentions allow us to recognise where we are in the moment, and being present and aware in that moment, embracing the journey more than the result.

Intentions focus on *attitudes* instead of *outcomes* and accomplishments. The problem with outcomes is that you do not have absolute control over what eventually materialises. For example, you can work hard but you may not necessarily get that promotion, so resolving to get a promotion this year is risky business.

Lack of self-judgement has to be worked at. It doesn't come naturally to most of us. In our professions, self-flagellation is nearly a prerequisite for the job.

How many of you have managed to keep your New Year resolutions? How many of you remember what your resolutions for this year are? How many of you have found joy and fulfilment because you kept your New Year resolutions?

I posed these questions to a group in a whole-practice seminar recently and I met with a communal shoulder hunch. What a ridiculous question to put to anyone in November. What an ineffectual method of raising morale.

Maybe my methods seem counterintuitive, but I had a reason for asking these questions quickly before the Christmas festivities set in, festivities which usually include indulgence.

Indulgence is often judged as 'wrong' and interchangeable with 'over-indulgence', also judged as 'wrong'.

Mental Wellbeing and Positive Psychology for Veterinary Professionals: A Pre-emptive, Proactive and Solution-based Approach, First Edition. Laura Woodward.
© 2024 John Wiley & Sons Ltd. Published 2024 by John Wiley & Sons Ltd.

'Decadent', 'naughty', 'forbidden' are all words used to describe chocolate and wine. Or, if you attend weight reduction organisations, 'syns' (supposedly short for synergistic, but let's be realistic). Other 'sins' include crisps, nuts and even bananas (only if mashed) and avocados (formerly known as super-foods).

It is this habitual tendency to be judgemental which makes us categorise foods, drinks, experiences, feelings, weather patterns, etc. as right or wrong. Mindful living has a huge emphasis on being non-judgemental, as we discussed in previous chapters. If we free ourselves of the constant necessity to judge things, situations, other people, our emotions, etc., we become liberated and a weight is lifted off our shoulders.

Because we have spent most of our lives categorising our experiences into good and bad boxes, it takes a lot of effort to break that habit. Only by consciously focusing on being non-judgemental for a few minutes at a time and then longer and longer can we begin to feel that relief. The good feelings which come from that liberation become the reward and the impetus to continue with the non-judgement. It takes effort and has to be a conscious decision.

So, what does this have to do with my resolution to have a dry January or lose two stone by March? Well, in making our New Year resolutions, the very thing we were hoping to gain by setting them – improved self-confidence, better liver function or a healthier body – can often become even more out of our reach when we 'fail' and then give up.

For example, by breaking my resolution to have a dry January, after one glass of wine, I may as well finish the bottle because once the resolution's broken there's no going back, right? Or, now that I've had two biscuits, I may as well have a tub of ice cream too, because I'm a failure at this.

And, come the end of January, I haven't lost a pound, so there's no way I'll be slimmer by June. Maybe I'll try again next year.

Now, not only have I achieved nothing I wanted to achieve, I've actually damaged my self-confidence even further and brought my mood to an even lower level than it was when I made the resolutions in the first place.

Not everyone is in this position. For some, January 1st brings a fresh target each year which is achieved and exceeded, and their self-esteem rises as a result. I am not in this cohort and so I propose a different way of setting goals this coming year.

New Year Intentions

An intention to do something means we can't fail. For example, if I make a New Year intention to drink less, then, every evening I drink less than I used to, I have 'made it', got a result, kept my intention, achieved my goal.

Similarly, if I go out to the pub and down a few pints of cheap lager, I haven't failed to the point where I may as well give up, binge the next night and restart the self-flagellation. I've simply drunk more than I intend to drink every night this year.

It's hard to fail at an intention. Every night I achieve my intention can be seen as a win *if I choose*.

Every time we carry out our intention, we have achieved something worthwhile. If we resolve to cut down on eating (as opposed to losing 10 kg), then, every time we deny ourselves a bag of crisps and every time we don't buy a bar of chocolate at the corner shop, we have succeeded. The reward can be instant if you allow it. Seems a bit airy fairy? Because success breeds more success, it may be the reason why you succeed this year where you didn't last year (or the year before that). Losing weight is the by-product of changing our attitude. Changing your attitude is the real success and something you do have control over.

If I eat two biscuits, I've eaten two biscuits. Lack of self-kindness could mean that this two-biscuit event would spiral into finishing the packet because I'm such a failure and such a resolution breaker, I don't deserve to be healthier or slimmer.

Body shaming is outdated and vile, yet we body shame ourselves daily. If only slim people went on the beach, we'd be living in Rio. Eating biscuits doesn't change your worthiness to breathe sea air and make sandcastles. Only you do that to yourself.

With a calmer, less judgemental mindset, I can be more logical and less urgent in my approach. Two biscuits are less likely to affect my mood than 20 biscuits. Therefore, instead of the self-destructive behaviours of last year, I can just stop there and see how I get on the next day.

Without the huge sense of failure which inevitably follows on from the breaking of a resolution, the morning after an evening where I drink the whole bottle can be a new day where the intention is the same.

In order to be less self-critical, it has to be a conscious decision. Sometimes, when we fail, the self-loathing that we habitually feel can lead us to 'punish' ourselves for bingeing by (you've guessed it) bingeing some more.

At the turn of the twentieth century, the Anti-Saloon League formed and persuaded its members to pledge their eternal sobriety to develop better character and set a good example. Falling off the wagon became a phrase used when someone who had made such a pledge had a drink. These days, a person using the phrase 'falling off the wagon' is possibly someone who subconsciously wants to 'fail' as an excuse to abandon the resolution and continue as before. It could also be used by someone who has lost all confidence in their ability to keep their resolutions after years of low achievement, and is ashamed of that fact because they presume others judge them as harshly as they judge themselves for 'failing'.

> This year I intend to be less self-berating when I inevitably do something which I would have previously judged as 'wrong'.

I recently talked with Matt, a vet from a large corporate practice. He said that he used to be a 'chaser'. For most of his life, he chased happiness, perfection and prosperity, frequently using the mindset 'if only I (had the perfect job, had enough money, had the perfect marriage)' or 'when I (lose 10 kg, get that promotion, find a girlfriend)'.

Every year, he would make a New Year resolution connected to one of his 'chases' – I will resolve to work out every day; I will start looking for a new job; I will join online dating – in an effort to finally feel fulfilled and satisfied in his life. He was always successful out of the gate but one setback would spiral him out of control and by February, he felt defeated and a New Year resolution failure, contributing to his sadness and depression.

Sound familiar?

If your New Year intention is to spend 10 minutes or more in mindful meditation in the morning, once you've done it the first time, it feels like a real start. Twice and you've set a precedent. Three times and it's become your new normal, a habit, part of your regular morning routine which you just do without questioning and you've achieved your goal already because the goal was to meditate, not to become a monk by March.

Because now the alarm is set for the same time each morning, you have intentionally 'created time' for yourself to benefit from however many minutes you've decided upon.

If you skip a day, it doesn't mean you've failed, it means you've skipped a day. It doesn't undo the previous day's work or negate its benefits. It doesn't mean you can't meditate tomorrow. It's not a failure. It's a skipped day.

I met another person in counselling, Julie, a nurse, who felt that everything in her life was determined by her size. If she put on weight, she felt that everyone judged her to be a rubbish nurse, a useless wife, a stupid waste of an ever-increasing space. She chased the dream of being thin and therefore successful.

Every January, Julie resolved to lose two stone that year. Every February she had already 'failed' and given up on herself. And yet, by February, she still had 11 months to lose the weight. The fact was that it only took one 'bad' day for Julie to give up on the only acceptable outcome for her. And that was it until the next New Year.

She joined Slimming World. But every time she put on weight, she was too embarrassed to turn up to the meetings. She would binge at night and wake up in the morning wondering who that person was who had eaten all the biscuits in the tin.

So profound was her self-loathing that if she ate one biscuit, it was such a failure in her mind that she binged on the rest of the packet. She had 'fallen off the wagon' by eating a biscuit, the forbidden fruit, a 'sin' and therefore what was the point in even trying?

If Julie had made a New Year intention to eat as few biscuits as she possibly could, rather than a resolution to lose two stone, then falling off the wagon wouldn't be a possibility, there would be no room for self-flagellation and the binges would become a rarity. Because, even eating one biscuit less than she wanted to would be an achievement in itself, no matter whether it was the last biscuit in the box or not.

The aim is to change our mindset and exert a degree of change as opposed to racing towards the ultimate goal of two stone weight loss from the day we take the Christmas tree down.

So Julie and I practised mindfulness-based eating awareness therapy (MBEAT) with dark chocolate digestives. Encouraging Julie to eat the one thing she was trying to banish from her life seemed counterintuitive, calorie-laden and contrary to what she had been doing every previous January for as long as she could remember.

We looked at the biscuits, carefully examining the wrinkled dark sheen on the chocolate side and the many different colours of light brown biscuit grains on the other. We slowly inhaled the mouth-watering, contrasting aromas of bitter chocolate and oaty biscuit.

The crunch of the first bite was the first time Julie had 'listened' to a biscuit (understandable, really). We felt the contrast between the two sides of the piece in our mouths and munched slowly, enjoying the mingling of the bitter and sweet tastes and then swallowed, enjoying the feeling of this treat starting to fill our bellies. It wasn't long before the sugar hit happened and it was gorgeous.

We must have spent a good 10 minutes eating that biscuit which Julie declared was the best biscuit she had ever eaten. She didn't fancy or need another to be satiated.

Julie applied this mindset to her daily life. She managed to eat half a pack of crisps most days. I can't do that. But more importantly, she did it without feeling that she had 'sinned'. Every time she left the rest of the crisps in the bag, she became stronger, admired herself a bit more, felt more compassionate towards herself. By exerting some self-compassion, we rid ourselves of the need to self-flagellate in the form of bingeing and abusing our useless, undisciplined bodies.

Not surprisingly, Julie lost a load of weight last year. More importantly, she judged herself less harshly and was able to appreciate that others were not relating her size to her worth as a nurse, wife and friend.

> When we cultivate a sense of caring and self-kindness towards ourselves, when we subsequently fail or experience shortcomings, instead of self-judgement and criticism, we build resilience that can contribute to motivation and lasting change.

Hence, when we stray off the path of our intention, if we learn from the experience, identify the triggers which push us off the path and get back on the path without self-deprecation, it builds more resilience every single time. These are the ways we keep the good intentions running at full throttle for the whole 12 months.

Postponing Mindfulness and Self-compassion

> *Happiness is not ready made. It comes from our own actions.*
>
> Dalai Lama

Chaos can be the impetus for us to start, rather than the excuse for us to procrastinate.

'I don't have the time', 'I'm just too tired' are some of the reasons why establishing a daily mindfulness practice is totally out of the question for now, no matter how convinced I am that it would be beneficial.

'Not yet.' 'Once things settle down.' We'll do it then.

Instead of waiting endlessly for the perfect time to start a daily mindfulness practice, we could instead just start.

Work is insanely busy and all-consuming. You might feel that you're being pulled in so many different directions you must resemble a large splat of paint. But the longer you leave it to start, the more work you will have to do to reach a place of peace.

As one patient of mine so beautifully put it after I introduced her to mindful breathing when mid-crisis, 'It's like I put a big tennis net in front of my snowball and stopped it getting bigger and faster down the hill'.

If you have no time, that's okay, you can incorporate mindful living into your life without stopping to sit on the cushion.

If you're too tired, remember that mindfulness helps insomnia and energises us. No, really. It's prescribed to people who want to stop temazepam but need a substitute which enables good-quality sleep. It works. It doesn't need to be done at bedtime. In fact, paradoxically, meditation helps insomnia even more if it's *not* done at bedtime.

If you fall asleep while meditating, do it first thing in the morning with a coffee in your hand sitting upright on the floor instead.

You may have great intentions, which work seamlessly on a quiet day. But what would be ideal is for you to practise mindfulness even on the days when you've forgotten to wash your child's PE kit, when the washing machine's just flooded the kitchen, the cat's vomited everywhere, when the tube is delayed and even when you have a hangover. You won't know until you try. So here are six steps to help you to start.

1) *Establish what you want to do and why you want to do it.* For example, it may be that you want to explore what mindfulness is all about on a personal level. Maybe you want to have more strength in a crisis, maybe you want to be more present so that you can roll with the punches of life and enjoy the sun when it shines. You decide why you want to do this. Write the reasons down.

2) *Make a non-negotiable schedule.* Many people find it easiest to meditate first thing in the morning before anyone else is awake. That involves getting up earlier. It sounds counterintuitive when you're already exhausted. Let me tell you a story. When I first began meditation, I was taught by a Sri Lankan Buddhist monk in Letchworth Garden City. It is a very purist form of meditation and mindfulness. My mentor, Bhante Samitha, told me to set my alarm half an hour earlier than normal every morning for my meditation. I dutifully did this and was so proud of myself, I reported back to him with pride. His calm reply was to tell me to set my alarm an *hour* earlier than normal instead. I followed his instructions and was leaping out of bed at 5 a.m. every morning full of excitement about meditating in the dark when most people were still asleep. Again, I reported back to him about how well I was doing. He was pleased and said I should get up at 4.30 and meditate for an hour and a half each morning. I did this and the story continues as you would expect. The day he said I should get up at 4 a.m. to meditate, I drew the line. No way. We both belly laughed till we cried. Now I know that 60 minutes is my own personal limit and 5 a.m. is my ideal time to start.

My point is that, as someone who loves sleep and needs sleep, as someone who has had problems with insomnia since I was at uni, I now wake up refreshed at 5 a.m. every morning with excitement. It's *my* non-negotiable schedule made by me for me. That's why it's valid and why I can stick to it.

It's not a competition. If 20 minutes is someone's scheduled non-negotiable daily practice, that's more helpful than postponing the schedule indefinitely.

Daily practice, even if for a very short time, is more beneficial than three hours one day and nothing for the rest of the week.

Just start. I suggest you start with 20 minutes every morning and then make your own non-negotiable schedule for yourself. By setting your alarm for 20 minutes before anyone else gets up, you are 'creating time'. So, no need to feel guilty for indulging yourself instead of pleasing others. No need to feel you should be checking emails or the progress of your inpatients overnight. This is bonus time you have made for this. It's non-negotiable. Nobody can do this for you, except you.

3) *Choose meditation or a mindful activity or a mixture.* Meditation doesn't suit everyone. Mindful activity with normal alarm times might be better for you. The object is to make it non-negotiable and feasible for you. Every time you brush your teeth, you could breathe mindfully for two minutes, focusing on only your breath. Sounds easy, right? That's another four minutes per day. Every second counts. If it's difficult, that's a fantastic opportunity to recognise that you're learning something new and wonderful.

Possibly, you'll choose to walk the dog mindfully with your phone off. Just being present, immersing yourself in the sounds, smells, temperature and sights around you. You can see it as multitasking for your benefit. You're walking the dog anyway. Now it can be for you as well as for your dog.

Maybe you can take 10 deep breaths each and every time you reach for your phone before you look at it. These days when we're getting our BBC news 'fix' hourly, posting on Facebook and Instagram and BeRealing at least once daily, that's going to be a significantly frequent time of calm. You could try it now for the next hour.

Mindful tea pouring, tea drinking and cup washing. Yes, it's all recognised mindfulness.

One of my favourites is mindful driving. The music is a yoga and meditation playlist from Spotify, my breathing is quiet and regular, my driving is smooth. I welcome other drivers to come in front of me and I thank them for thanking me. All very hippy. After a noisy crazy day at work, half an hour of driving home like that and I'm in the zone, de-stressed and calm.

4) *Make a mindfulness hub.* Making a welcoming place where you can practise makes it more likely that you'll do it. Perhaps you can use a

comfy cushion, some incense and headphones. Maybe an eye mask, maybe some quiet music. If it's all left *in situ*, you're ready to go.

5) *Decide in advance what you're going to do.* Maybe you have a list of guided meditations and you've decided which one you're going to do each day. Maybe you can write down one thing you want to focus on while doing unguided meditation each day for the next few days.
   Meditation isn't some magic trance only experts can achieve. Simply put, it's a bit of a breather for your brain.

6) *Notice non-judgementally.* Some days, it will feel like you can reach the 'zone' immediately. As soon as you close your eyes you are 'seeing' with your 'third eye' on the bridge of your nose, between your real eyes. Other days, maybe you won't be in that place at all. Remember, even monks have days when they find it difficult to meditate.

   If it's a great day for mindfulness, notice the success and enjoy. If it's a rubbish day for mindfulness, notice the frustration or difficulty. The important thing is to notice non-judgementally, i.e. no self-flagellation, no yearning for it to be different, no berating yourself for being 'bad' at mindfulness and meditation.

   Our success is in noticing that we didn't succeed in the way we had originally planned, and accepting the emotions which ensue.

   Also *noticing* the difficulty means you have started incorporating mindfulness into your life, which can bring you a sense of pride and accomplishment.

When you're quiet, everything settles on the floor of your mind like sediment in undisturbed still water.

Megan Monahan

Index